16 weeks to
achieve your goal
of a healthy lifestyle

The Never SayDiet

Personal Fitness Trainer

Chantel Hobbs

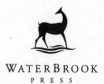

WATERBROOK
PRESS

THE NEVER SAY DIET PERSONAL FITNESS TRAINER
PUBLISHED BY WATERBROOK PRESS
12265 Oracle Boulevard, Suite 200
Colorado Springs, Colorado 80921

This book is not intended as a substitute for the advice and care of your physician, and as with any other fitness, diet, or nutrition plan, you should use proper discretion, in consultation with your physician, in utilizing the information presented. The author and the publisher expressly disclaim responsibility for any adverse effects that may result from the use or application of the information contained in this book.

All Scripture quotations, unless otherwise indicated, are taken from the Holy Bible, New International Version®. NIV®. Copyright © 1973, 1978, 1984 by International Bible Society. Used by permission of Zondervan Publishing House. All rights reserved. Scripture quotations marked (NLT) are taken from the Holy Bible, New Living Translation, copyright © 1996. Used by permission of Tyndale House Publishers Inc., Wheaton, Illinois 60189. All rights reserved.

ISBN 978-0-307-44642-8

Published in the United States by WaterBrook Multnomah, an imprint of the Crown Publishing Group, a division of Random House Inc., New York.

Library of Congress Cataloging-in-Publication Data
Hobbs, Chantel.
   The never say diet personal fitness trainer: 16 weeks to achieve your goal of a healthy lifestyle / Chantel Hobbs. — 1st ed.
       p. cm.
   Includes bibliographical references.
   Summary: "After losing 200 pounds, a mother of four reveals her straightforward, no-excuses program for permanent weight loss and complete life change—involving mind, body, and spirit."—Provided by publisher.
   ISBN 978-0-307-44642-8
   1. Weight loss. 2. Reducing exercises. 3. Physical fitness. I. Title.
   RM222.2.H574 2008
   613.2'5—dc22

                                    2008039501

Printed in the United States of America
2010

10 9 8 7 6 5 4 3

Contents

Phase 4: Get Strong (Weeks 13–16)

Do You Have Enough Desire?

Did you know that several days before the Super Bowl, T-shirts are printed announcing the winner of the game? Here's how it works: the official NFL apparel companies create shirts naming each team as the winner and then produce both versions. Immediately after the game, they sell the correct T-shirts and donate the losers' shirts to World Vision, a Christian organization that does relief and development work in impoverished countries.

According to Worldvision.com, somewhere in Africa a man is wearing a T-shirt celebrating the New England Patriots as the winner of the 2008 Super Bowl.[1] At the same time, a New York Giants fan who is reading this is hyperventilating, maybe even taking the Patriots' name in vain!

I am more the party planner than a spectator for the annual Super Bowl event at our house, but the match-up between the Giants and Patriots was memorable even for me. With the Patriots favored to win after an undefeated season, the Giants surprised us with a legendary win. How did the underdog defeat the obvious favorite? It wasn't magical Gatorade or flashier uniforms. The Giants achieved greatness through superior coaching, determination, and the decision not to give up or give in. No one could have predicted which team would have the most intense will to win the big game, but after four quarters we all knew.

Sure, the New England Patriots thought they had it sewn up. But they hadn't bargained on the smothering defense of the under-dog New York Giants—the team that came to win and make foot-ball history!

Here is what Super Bowl XLII has to do with you. It's time to start your new life, and it's no exaggeration to say you can make your own history. Right now you might not have a lot of confidence when it comes to losing weight and getting fit. You have probably tried to lose weight many times in the past and failed, just like I did. I eventually accepted that I had to live in a state of depression, sure that nothing would ever click.

But finally I "got" the fact that God wanted me to have a much better, much healthier life. That was part of His will for me, and I could join my will to His. He and I both wanted me to become the best I could be each day. I realized that becoming thinner and healthier was a spiritual journey. The odds of trying again and *winning* this time were on my side, because I chose to win the battle one day at a time with God.

Over the past several years, I have learned that to be the cham-pion of your health and fitness, you must have a clear direction and a committed heart, nothing more and nothing less. You are training for a new life, so forget the defeats of the past. Begin today to believe that you can change, and pledge that this time is the last time.

The Never Say Diet Personal Fitness Trainer delivers a sixteen-week plan that puts into practice the diet and fitness secrets from my book *Never Say Diet.* Each week begins with inspiration from the Word of God, an inspiring quote, and a jolt of motivation. We will pursue nutrition, exercise, fitness, and weight loss in a way that is doable. You'll be excited as you begin to see results within a few weeks. This book will help train your body, your mind, and your spirit. Remember, the process of getting fit and changing your life is a spiritual battle!

This book provides space for journaling. Since this is your *new* life we're working on, keeping track of your progress will create a record that will be fun to look back on! (If you like to add a lot of detail in your writing, keep a spiral notebook handy so you'll have plenty of space.) Before the sixteen weeks are over, you will lose weight, become seriously fit, and feel confident about your future!

As you use *The Never Say Diet Personal Fitness Trainer,* you will receive emotional support, practical advice on nutrition and exercise, and daily help in relying on God and trusting that He wants what is best for you. Addressing mind, body, and spirit—all three—is the key to bringing about permanent change. (This book is a companion to *Never Say Diet,* so keep a copy of *Never Say Diet* close at hand to use as a reference.)

Week by week we will tackle your program together, and you will enjoy the thrill of accomplishment as you achieve one goal at a time, one day at a time. Bring your desire, let God be the driving force, and I will be your coach! It's time to make your own history.

Before we begin this focused diet and exercise program, I advise you to first consult your physician. When I created the program in *Never Say Diet*—the program we're following in this book—I worked closely with experts in medicine, nutrition, and physiology. The program is sound, but still, you should see your personal physician before beginning this or any nutrition, exercise, and fitness program.

Also consider using *The Never Say Diet Personal Fitness Trainer* with a few friends or in your small group. You can find a leader's discussion guide at www.chantelhobbs.com.

Get a Move On!

Weeks 1–4

The Perfect Body Type: Yours!

You Are Lovely Today

Scripture for the week: "I praise you because I am fearfully and wonderfully made; your works are wonderful, I know that full well.... When I was woven together in the depths of the earth, your eyes saw my unformed body."

—PSALM 139:14–16

Quote for the week: "Faith, as Paul saw it, was a living, flaming thing leading to surrender and obedience to the commandments of Christ."

—A. W. TOZER

As you begin the journey to never say *diet,* remember that your value is based on who you are in Christ, not what the number on the scale says. God created everything about you, and He knows you better than you know yourself. He knows which foods are your weaknesses, and He is there whenever the temptation to overeat or consume unhealthy food seems overwhelming.

The Lord knows the tears you have shed out of desperation. He was there to comfort you when it seemed like no one understood your pain. Trust me, on days when I feel the most flawed, I need the verses from Psalm 139 to remind me of what is true. The living God formed every part of my body, even the parts I would like to change.

Although I used to struggle and fail in caring for my body, God always knew it best. When I finally cried out to my Creator and invited Him to help with the repair, I knew I could succeed. He wants you to succeed too.

Start this week by thanking the Lord for the gifts of your life and your body. By focusing on making some improvements, you will ultimately be honoring Him more and more each day.

Find a recent photo of yourself, or take one, and tape it in the space that follows. This picture will be a powerful reference for you in the coming weeks as you begin your transformation.

THE MIND FACTOR: CHANGE YOUR BRAIN

In *Never Say Diet*, I make a big deal about the Five Decisions—and for good reason. You will fail in this new attempt to change your life unless you first change your brain. To succeed, you need to be willing to do whatever it takes—unconditionally. I want to be your cheerleader and your friend. And for us to get going, you need to commit to the five Brain Change decisions found on pages 76–82 of *Never Say Diet*.

Think about how each of the Five Decisions applies to your life. Also, try to memorize them. They will form the backbone you need to stand up to and overcome every area of weakness in your life. Create your personal surrender statement.

THE EXERCISE EQUATION: ARE YOU WILLING?

This week your first assignment is to start building a foundation of discipline. You will be successful over the next month if you show up for exercise thirty minutes a day, five days in a row, every week—*no matter what.* There are many choices for your cardiovascular exercise. Below is a list of suggestions. Even if your week gets hectic, finding the time to make this happen is *imperative.*

Cardio Exercise Suggestions

Basketball	Spinning class
Bike riding	Stair climber
Cross-country skiing machine	Stair stepper
Dancing	Stationary bike/ recumbent bike
Elliptical machine	Step aerobics
Jogging/running	Swimming
Kick boxing	Tennis
Racquetball	Walking

How to Take Your Measurements

Taking your measurements at the beginning of each month is an important part of the process of losing weight. You will begin to see precisely where you are losing fat. As you start building more muscle, there will be months where your progress is more evident in your measurements than on the scale, because muscle is denser than fat.

You will begin by taking six measurements. You should be able to do them by yourself, with the exception of your upper arm. (Ask a friend or your spouse to help you.) For instructions on taking accurate measurements, see pages 97–98 of *Never Say Diet.* Record your measurements below.

Bust: _____

Chest: _____

Waist: _____

Hips: _____

Thighs: _____

Arms: _____

Be sure that you consistently measure in the same spots each month. I also recommend taking your measurements *before* your workouts.

Weigh Yourself

Weigh yourself, and record your weight at the beginning of each week. Week 1 starting weight: _____

WEEK 1 CARDIO TRAINING

Complete your cardio exercise five days in a row, for at least thirty minutes per day. In the space provided, write down the day, the date, the exercise you completed, and the duration of each exercise period. This serves as a reminder that you always found a way to get the exercise done, whether you felt like it or not.

Day 1 date/exercise/duration:

_____

How did it go?

_____

Day 2 date/exercise/duration:

_____

How did it go?

_____

Day 3 date/exercise/duration:

_____

How did it go?

_____

Day 4 date/exercise/duration:

_____

How did it go?

_____

Day 5 date/exercise/duration:

_____

How did it go?

_____

The Food Factor: Breakfast Is Where It's At

This week you must place your nutritional focus on the most important meal of the day: breakfast. Plan to eat every day within two
hours of waking up. Listed below are some fresh food ideas. Each
one is about three hundred calories, which is perfect!

- Quaker Weight Control oatmeal, 1 tablespoon of raisins,
  cinnamon to taste, 2 slices of turkey bacon.
- One slice of whole-wheat toast, light spread of peanut
  butter (natural is best), and ½ grapefruit.
- Chocolate strawberry shake. Blend the following: 1 scoop
  chocolate protein powder, 10 small frozen strawberries,
  1 packet sugar substitute, ½ cup low-fat milk, a few ice
  cubes.
- Egg white omelet. In a skillet with nonstick spray, cook veg-
  gies you like, 3 lightly beaten egg whites, and 1 tablespoon
  fat-free cheese. Accompany with half an English muffin with
  a dab of peanut butter.

Each of these breakfast meals provides a good balance of protein,
carbs, and fat. This ensures your day gets off to a good start; it is
igniting your source of energy. Find a few meals that you enjoy, and
keep repeating them. This way you won't stress out over deciding
what to have.

Week 1 Breakfast Log

Using the space provided, record each day's breakfast menu and the
portions.

Day 1 date/time: _____

_____

Day 2 date/time: _____

_____

Day 3 date/time: _____

_____

Day 4 date/time: _____

_____

Day 5 date/time: _____

_____

Day 6 date/time: _____

_____

Day 7 date/time: _____

_____

Dare to Be Disciplined

Understand Your Part—and God's Part

Scripture for the week: "Do you not know that in a race all the runners run, but only one gets the prize? Run in such a way as to get the prize. Everyone who competes in the games goes into strict training. They do it to get a crown that will not last; but we do it to get a crown that will last forever."

—1 CORINTHIANS 9:24–25

Quote for the week: "Christian, remember the goodness of God in the frost of adversity."

—CHARLES SPURGEON

When I was a little girl, sometimes discipline meant getting a little whack with my daddy's homemade paddle. I was a serious drama queen, the child who screamed hysterically before the paddle even touched her behind. As much as I feared it, looking back now, I can see that the discipline came out of my parents' love and their desire for me to learn obedience. However, it sure didn't seem like it at the time.

Years later, when I committed to making my health and fitness a priority, I began by viewing my training program as harsh discipline. I viewed the treadmill as punishment for the poor job I had done taking care of my body in the past.

However, in a short time discipline took on a completely different meaning. It became a training tool—something I wanted to master and benefit from. No longer did I view healthy eating and exercise as punishment. Just the opposite: they were privileges. If you focus on becoming a disciplined person, you will realize this is the foundation for all your successes in life.

THE MIND FACTOR: MAKING EXCUSES ONLY BUYS DISAPPOINTMENT

The anticipation and excitement of seeing yourself thinner and more fit can dwindle in a few days when "real life" takes over. So this week you can't allow yourself any wiggle room. Don't even consider the option of falling back on a convenient excuse. The training plan won't work unless you stick to your commitments.

When you're cooking and you want to make sure what you're preparing comes out perfectly, you move the pot to the front burner. Because getting fit and staying fit will *always* be a priority in your life, you need to be careful not to let it slide to the back burner. Maybe an overcrowded schedule, a business trip, or a family crisis makes you think you should hold off for a better time. If you're tempted to put things off, remind yourself of this truth: there is no better time than now to change your life.

It's easy to allow the hectic pace of life to become an excuse. I used to lie to myself by saying, "There aren't enough hours in the day." I also felt like I was too far gone to change. But really, how could I have been too busy to take care of myself? How could I think that I was past the point of no return when I know how big God is? So make a commitment right now: I will not allow any of my old excuses to distract me.

THE EXERCISE EQUATION: DRINK IT UP

Now that you have completed a full week of regular exercise, you may feel some soreness, or you may find that you get tired a little earlier in the day. As your body becomes more accustomed to working out, not only will this go away, but you will begin to feel better than you have in a long time. In all five of your weekly workouts, be sure you are breaking a sweat. As you exercise, keep your mind on what you're doing. Focus on the exercise goal for the month: you are training yourself to practice discipline, which means you no longer buy your old excuses.

Discipline for this month means:

• You will make time in your schedule, no matter what comes up.
• You will show up each day and move for thirty minutes, elevating your heart rate and breaking a sweat.
• You will avoid the trap of focusing on your weight.
• You will know you have succeeded when you are consistent in showing up.

Don't forget that when you sweat, you lose fluid. Use this formula to calculate the amount of water you need to drink to keep yourself hydrated: divide your body weight (in pounds) by two. This is the number of ounces of water you need to drink daily. (If you weigh 130 pounds, drink 65 ounces of water per day, or eight 8-ounce glasses.)

Weigh Yourself

Record your weight at the beginning of this week.

Week 2 starting weight: _____ (gain or loss of _____ pounds)

WEEK 2 CARDIO TRAINING

Record in the space provided what kind of cardio exercise you did and the duration of each day's exercise. Also this week record your water intake.

Day 1 date/exercise/duration:

_____

Ounces of water consumed today: _____
How did it go?

_____

Day 2 date/exercise/duration:

_____

Ounces of water consumed today: _____
How did it go?

_____

Day 3 date/exercise/duration:

_____

Ounces of water consumed today: _____
How did it go?

_____

Day 4 date/exercise/duration:

_____

Ounces of water consumed today: _____
How did it go?

_____

Day 5 date/exercise/duration:

_____

Ounces of water consumed today: _____
How did it go?

_____

The Food Factor: Hungry or Not, Fill the Tank

Most people who skip breakfast tell me it's because they aren't hungry when they first wake up. You need to ask yourself which scenario makes more sense: would you rather put gas in your car when there is still some fuel in the tank or wait until you are running on fumes?

You don't want to leave home in the morning and immediately start running on fumes. Commit to eating breakfast every morning. It will give you the boost necessary to crank your engine and get the most out of your day.

As you choose what to eat, think about the importance of protein. It's easy to shortchange protein at breakfast, especially if you're like me and don't enjoy eggs. (And most people are not drawn to a piece of chicken or grilled fish in the morning.) However, you need to include protein at breakfast. It will make you feel full for a longer period of time than eating mostly carbohydrates.

Following are some high-protein breakfast foods. Try fitting one of these into your breakfast meal each day this week.

Cottage cheese

Eggs/egg whites/Egg Beaters

Healthy Choice ham or other low-fat, low-sodium lunchmeat

Peanut butter

A shake made with protein powder, either soy or whey

Turkey bacon

Yogurt

Week 2 Breakfast Log

Record each day's breakfast menu, including protein items, and the portions.

Day 1 date/time: _____

_____

Day 2 date/time: _____

_____

Day 3 date/time: _____

_____

Day 4 date/time: _____

_____

Day 5 date/time: _____

_____

Day 6 date/time: _____

_____

Day 7 date/time: _____

_____

Who's the Boss?

Ask God to Be

Scripture for the week: "Praise be to the LORD, for he has heard my cry for mercy. The LORD is my strength and my shield; my heart trusts in him, and I am helped."

—PSALM 28:6–7

Quote for the week: "You can do anything if you have enthusiasm. Enthusiasm is the yeast that makes your hopes rise to the stars. With it, there is accomplishment. Without it there are only alibis."

—HENRY FORD

Have you ever needed some serious mercy? I have. When I have been at the lowest points in my life, crying out to God for mercy felt like the only thing I could do. When we ask for mercy, we are seeking compassion and forgiveness. This is what God does best!

When it comes to your weaknesses and past mistakes, God simply wants you to trust Him more. We could have more joy than we know what to do with if we would remind ourselves where our strength comes from. Meeting your weight-loss goals will be easier if you draw on God's bigness and His ability to shield you from temptation.

THE MIND FACTOR: ENTHUSIASM EQUALS ENERGY

This week you will start to experience the benefits of pursuing a new life. You will feel more alive, like you're waking up in a special way. You will also notice that the challenges don't stop just because you're making progress.

The world is full of people who seem bent on stealing everyone else's joy. I try to protect myself, so I limit the time I spend watching television news. You can't control the world, but you can control whether you let outside influences affect you. As you enter the third week, begin each day by committing that you will allow nothing and no one to put you in a bad mood. Take the initiative to put positive people in your life. Then draw encouragement and enthusiasm from them.

THE EXERCISE EQUATION: WHY A SCHEDULE MATTERS

This week find a set time every day to do your workout. You should complete thirty minutes of exercise, five days in a row. In my work as a personal trainer for clients, I have found that a sporadic exercise time slot leads to disaster. Before you know it, the day can get away from you, and your best intentions end up unfulfilled.

If your life allows it, do your exercises first thing in the morning. But if that's impossible, don't beat yourself up. As long as you have a set time every day, you'll do fine. Begin to view those thirty minutes as a gift you give yourself. This can be your time to disappear from other obligations, burn calories, and reduce stress.

Working out early works for me because it guarantees that I have limited noise and distractions. Ask yourself when is the optimal time for you to exercise, and write that time in the space provided. Even if you need to vary the time slightly based on the day of the week, settle on it now and put it in writing.

My daily exercise time: _____

Weigh Yourself

Record your weight at the beginning of this week.

Week 3 starting weight: _____ (gain or loss of _____ pounds)

WEEK 3 CARDIO TRAINING

Record in the space provided what kind of cardio exercise you did and the duration of each day's exercise.

Day 1 date/exercise/duration:

_____

How did it go?

_____

Day 2 date/exercise/duration:

_____

How did it go?

_____

Day 3 date/exercise/duration:

_____

How did it go?

_____

Day 4 date/exercise/duration:

_____

How did it go?

_____

Day 5 date/exercise/duration:

_____

How did it go?

_____

THE FOOD FACTOR: SHAKE IT UP

Now that you're starting the third week, eating breakfast should be nearly automatic. And for the record, a cup of coffee will never count as breakfast!

If you've never tried a protein shake, have one this week. I'll give you two recipes that are quick and easy to make, and they really keep you satisfied.

Strawberry shortcake shake. Blend 1 scoop vanilla or strawberry protein powder, 6 frozen strawberries, ½ low-fat graham cracker, ½ cup low-fat milk, and ½ cup water.

Chocolate-walnut-banana delight. Blend 1 scoop chocolate protein powder, ½ frozen banana, 8 whole walnuts, ½ cup low-fat milk, ½ cup water, and 5 ice cubes.

Feel free to experiment with similar ingredients. When purchasing protein powder, look for whey or soy. Each has its benefits, so you may want to try both.

Week 3 Breakfast Log

Continue to record your breakfast meals. It's important to include protein in the menu. And this week, don't fail to recognize and celebrate your success! Write down the day, date, and time of day, then the menu and portions.

Day 1 date/time: _____

_____

Day 2 date/time: _____

_____

Day 3 date/time: _____

_____

Day 4 date/time: _____

_____

Day 5 date/time: _____

_____

_____

Day 6 date/time: _____

_____

Day 7 date/time: _____

_____

God's Property

Don't Forget: You've Been Paid For!

Scripture for the week: "Do you not know that your body is a temple of the Holy Spirit, who is in you, whom you have received from God? You are not your own; you were bought at a price. Therefore honor God with your body."

—1 CORINTHIANS 6:19–20

Quote for the week: "Sweat plus sacrifice equals success."

—CHARLIE FINLEY

You might be wondering why I didn't use those verses from 1 Corinthians for Week 1. Here's why I waited. I wanted you to recognize that you are God's special, unique creation—and then remind you of the obligation we all have to our Creator. When we invite God to be the Lord of our lives, He dwells inside us. Even when we're not taking care of our health, He still lives in us.

For almost thirty years I failed to take care of my body. When I think about it now, I'm embarrassed that I entertained Jesus with filthy floors, laundry scattered around, and dirty dishes in the sink. That's a pretty accurate picture of the ways we neglect our bodies.

God has told us we are "wonderfully made,"[2] but even so we sometimes take our bodies for granted. As the initial excitement of losing weight and changing your body wears off, you'll find that it's more of a challenge to stay on track. Remind yourself that your body is a gift from God and that God dwells inside you. If your commitment to fitness starts to waver, let these facts renew your motivation to press on.

This week pray each day about your need to honor your Creator by giving Him a healthy place to dwell. Tell Him your desire to be a better "housekeeper" and to honor His creation—you!

The Mind Factor: Your First Peak Moment

I own a great T-shirt. It says, "I don't glisten, I sweat!" Some days when I think about the overweight and miserable me from years past, it makes me laugh to wear this shirt. I use to loathe sweating. The fact that I now enjoy sporting a shirt that has this message says a lot about my new life.

If you haven't already made some shifts in how you think about your body and your health, you will very soon. During this fourth week of your program, be thinking about the peak moment that is coming in a few days. You will have invested an entire month in your exercise regimen. You will have been committed and disciplined for four solid weeks! Congratulations!

I would guess there have been a few days when you thought *Who will know if I don't exercise today?* Or even, *How much could I possibly lose from just one workout?* When those temptations arise, you know that the commitment to become a better person is between you and God. You are not ultimately accountable to me, your spouse, or your best friend. You have surrendered your life to God. He will know if you give in to one of your old excuses. Measurable results are just around the corner. So press on and get ready to enter Phase 2 next week.

The Exercise Equation: Let's Kick It Up

You have almost completed Phase 1. You should be feeling strong and excited. At the beginning of this week, I want you to pick one day of your workout and do something to make it more intense by increasing your speed, adding ten minutes to the time period, or making the resistance more challenging.

If you are ambitious, do this for *two* of your exercise days. I can remember the end of the first month after I got started. I had an itch for a greater challenge. I spent the first month using only the recumbent bike at the gym. After a few weeks, I made a game out of seeing how long my heart and legs could handle more intensity. Each time I would do more, I felt a bit stronger. Plan to exit this month with a bang.

Weigh Yourself
Record your weight at the beginning of this week.

Week 4 starting weight: _____ (gain or loss of _____ pounds)

WEEK 4 CARDIO TRAINING

Record in the space provided what kind of cardio exercise you did and the duration of each day's exercise. Also, circle the one or two days where you "kicked it up."

Day 1 date/exercise/duration:

_____

How did it go?

_____

Day 2 date/exercise/duration:

_____

How did it go?

_____

Day 3 date/exercise/duration:

_____

How did it go?

_____

Day 4 date/exercise/duration:

_____

How did it go?

_____

Day 5 date/exercise/duration:

_____

How did it go?

_____

The Food Factor: Living La Vita Liquid

In *Never Say Diet* I describe our need to view food as fuel for our bodies. This can help break the thought pattern of *What am I in the mood for?* at each meal, a common mentality for an overweight person. The goal is to stop selecting what you eat based on gratification.

The *Never Say Diet* program is unique because it starts with the commitment to move five days in a row every week for the first month while pretty much leaving alone one's eating habits, other than breakfast. When I started this regimen, something strange occurred by the fourth week. I was beginning to crave healthier food and smaller portions without really trying. The way I was feeling on the inside, because I was sticking to my promise to exercise, began to help me in other ways. And best of all, it gave me hope for the future.

After holding to my initial commitments for four weeks, I then transformed my decision to get moving into a new commitment for greater achievements and weight loss. This week become aware of the calories you take in from what you are *drinking*. Consuming sodas, sweet tea, juices, and alcohol can be a main reason you have trouble losing weight.

Try cutting out calories that you drink, with the exception of protein shakes. If you are a soda drinker, try diet drinks or club soda with lemon. If you need a latte or coffee with sugar, use a sugar substitute.

Week 4 Breakfast Log

Continue to record your breakfast meals. Write down the day, date, and time of day on the first line, then the items and portions in the space below. This week add something new: in addition to the food you are eating, record the liquid calories you are *giving up*.

Day 1 date/time: _____

_____

Day 2 date/time: _____

_____

Day 3 date/time: _____

_____

Day 4 date/time: _____

_____

Day 5 date/time: _____

_____

Day 6 date/time: _____

_____

Day 7 date/time: _____

_____

_____

Take Charge!

Weeks 5–8

The Fruit Within

Self-Control Is Already Yours

Scripture for the week: "But the fruit of the Spirit is love, joy, peace, patience, kindness, goodness, faithfulness, gentleness and self-control."

—GALATIANS 5:22–23

Quote for the week: "Perseverance is the hard work you do after you get tired of doing the hard work you already did."

—NEWT GINGRICH

If you are a Christian, join me in giving up the expression "I have no self-control." I realize that everyone overindulges on occasion—with something. However, when we asked Jesus to take over our lives, we also invited the Holy Spirit to dwell inside us. This means we should be actively bearing the fruit of the Spirit, which includes self-control.

My grandparents once had several orange trees in their backyard. As a little girl who had a serious fascination with food, I thought it was fun to pick fruit off a branch and eat it immediately. (This was long before the pesticide problem!) I can remember there being a few trees that never had any oranges on them. Eventually, Pepa decided to cut them down. I can still hear him saying they were just "taking up space."

God put us on earth to bear fruit. My prayer is that I will never allow a day to go by when I am just "taking up space." Do you feel the same way? Ask God to help you make full use of the self-control that is already inside you.

THE MIND FACTOR: YOU GOTTA GIVE IT UP

Give it up! Three little words, and yet as I say them, I know they are scary. "Do you mean I have to give up my favorite things in life?" Maybe a few of them, if they involve overeating, inactivity, or taking your body for granted. "Do you mean I have to give up control over my life?" Only if you give God full control.

Now that you have completed Phase 1—Get a Move On!— you've seen the benefit of "giving it up." You have established a foundation of discipline with daily exercise. You have begun eating breakfast every morning, consuming a healthy amount of water, recording your ups and downs with exercise and nutrition. You have made all those changes in just four weeks, and we haven't even talked yet about weight loss or dropping a dress size.

Celebrate your progress as you enter Phase 2! You made the Five Decisions and established a foundation for a new life. Now it's time to build on the foundation. By following a reliable plan, we can do much more with our lives than we ever thought possible.

As you enter Phase 2 this week and add strength training to the mix, you may be uncomfortable in the beginning. Try to remember that all worthwhile things take practice to do well. By adding strength training and also giving up your food temptations for the next month, you start personalizing this program. This gives you ownership of your new lifestyle.

Each time you look temptation in the face and say no, you gain more strength. For me, it involved saying no to a cookie. I didn't say no to all cookies for all time, just one cookie at that moment. Then, the next time, I said no to the next cookie. It was one cookie at a time, one day at a time.

What is in your life that has some hold over you? What are you willing to give up?

THE EXERCISE EQUATION: THE STABILITY BALL AND YOU

This is going to be a fun and challenging week! Be sure to keep your copy of *Never Say Diet* close by as you start on strength training. This week you will begin to log both your cardio workouts and your strength training. The first thing you need to do is purchase a stability ball if you don't have one already. On my Web site, www.chantel hobbs.com, you can see the type of stability ball you need. Make sure you purchase the size that is appropriate for your height. (See page 113 in *Never Say Diet* to determine the right size ball for you.) Also, look to see that it says "stays in place" somewhere on the box.

As you work on strength training, stick it out even if it seems awkward at first. It will get easier.

It's Measurement Time

Measurements help you see exactly where you're slimming down, especially when the scale seems to fluctuate or to be totally stuck. First, copy your initial measurements from Week 1 in the space below. Then next to your old measurements, record this week's measurements. And next to that, calculate the difference. Don't be discouraged if the change isn't dramatic. As you establish better eating habits this month, your weight will drop more rapidly.

As you did before, take six measurements.

	Week 1	Week 5	Loss or Gain (in inches)
Bust:	_____	_____	_____
Chest:	_____	_____	_____
Waist:	_____	_____	_____
Hips:	_____	_____	_____
Thighs:	_____	_____	_____
Arms:	_____	_____	_____

Weigh Yourself

Record your weight at the beginning of this week.

Week 5 starting weight: _____ (gain or loss of _____ pounds)

Strength Training (2 Days, 20 Minutes per Session)

This first week of strength training you might not get far in completing all the exercises, but within a short time your flexibility and strength will improve. By recording your strength-training sessions, you have a place to reference your efforts, improvement, and peak moments. Be sure to take the challenges when you're ready—and don't forget to have a ball! (For descriptions of these exercises, refer to pages 115–24 in *Never Say Diet*.)

1. Bridge: 10 Reps, 1–2 Sets

Day 1: _____

_____

Day 2: _____

_____

2. Trunk Lift with Arm T: 10 Reps, 1–2 Sets

Day 1: _____

_____

Day 2: _____

_____

3. Alternating Hip Extension: 10 Reps, 1–2 Sets

Day 1: _____

_____

Day 2: _____

_____

4. Seated March: 10 Reps, 1–2 Sets

Day 1: _____

_____

Day 2: _____

_____

5. Seated Abdominal Walk Out: 10 Reps, 1–2 Sets

Day 1: _____

_____

Day 2: _____

_____

6. Seated Diagonal Reaches: 10 Reps, 1–2 Sets

Day 1: _____

_____

Day 2: _____

_____

7. Trunk Curl: 10 Reps, 1–2 Sets

Day 1: _____

_____

Day 2: _____

_____

8. Wall Squat: 10 Reps, 1–2 Sets

Day 1: _____

_____

Day 2: _____

_____

9. Wall Lunge: 10 Reps, 1–2 Sets

Day 1: _____

_____

Day 2: _____

_____

10. Wall Push-up: 10 Reps, 1–2 Sets

Day 1: _____

_____

Day 2: _____

_____

WEEK 5 CARDIO TRAINING

Complete thirty minutes of cardio exercises for five days this week, as you have in previous weeks. Record in the space provided what kind of cardio exercise you did and how it went.

Day 1 date/exercise/duration:

_____

How did it go?

_____

Day 2 date/exercise/duration:

_____

How did it go?

_____

Day 3 date/exercise/duration:

_____

How did it go?

_____

Day 4 date/exercise/duration:

_____

How did it go?

_____

Day 5 date/exercise/duration:

_____

How did it go?

_____

THE FOOD FACTOR: STOP BEFORE YOU FEEL FULL

You are going to approach each meal this week with the following attitude: *I do not need to feel completely satisfied to be satisfied.* Okay, I'm not going to lie to you. Doing this will be really hard for people with a compulsive personality. If something is good, we don't know when to stop. We think if a little of it is good, then more of it is even better.

To overcome this inclination, it's important to think of your body as a bank account. Calorie-wise, you have been giving your body much more than it needs, and your body has been nice enough to hold it for you. To handle the extra calories, it created a savings account. Think of this account as a "fat fund." Now is the time to tap into your "fat fund" and begin to use the stored-up calories.

Begin this new habit by walking away from the table while you still want a little more food. In other words, put the fork down sooner than you usually would. Remember, this month is not about changing all the foods you've been eating. Instead, you will cut back and tell yourself it's okay to be hungry for a bit. You won't die!

If pizza is on the menu, start with a big plate full of salad, and limit yourself to one slice of pizza. Use Week 5 as a special time to start addressing your biggest food weaknesses by staying clear of them. When you give up something, you are taking charge of your nutrition and asserting that food is losing its power over you! With sugar, pizza, chips, or any other food obsession, the more you have, the more you crave. As you eliminate certain foods, they no longer tempt you.

Week 5 Food Log

This week begin recording *everything* you eat—not just what you have for breakfast. Seeing it on paper will help you understand how much food you're consuming. It also will force you to pay closer attention to serving sizes and calorie content. Write down the day, date, and every item of food you consume each day.

Day 1: _____

_____

_____

_____

Day 2: _____

_____

_____

_____

Day 3: _____

_____

_____

_____

Day 4: _____

_____

_____

_____

Day 5: _____

_____

_____

_____

Day 6: _____

_____

_____

_____

Day 7: _____

_____

_____

The Ultimate Fighting Team: You and God

Where Does Your Strength Come From?

Scripture for the week: "I have learned the secret of being content in any and every situation, whether well fed or hungry, whether living in plenty or in want. I can do everything through him who gives me strength."

—PHILIPPIANS 4:12–13

Quote for the week: "Hard work spotlights the character of people: some turn up their sleeves, some turn up their noses, and some don't turn up at all."

—SAM EWING

What we need and what we want are two separate things. I recently picked out a Coach purse that I felt I *needed*. My husband, Keith, didn't *want* me to spend the money it would take to buy it. Just try to convince a man that an expensive purse provides *needed* entertainment value.

When it comes to choosing to eat less, the challenge is that we too often find ourselves in a state of want. As the verses in Philippians say, we can learn to be content in any circumstances. And remember, "I can do everything through him who gives me strength" (verse 13). Are you able to be content even in a state of want?

Eating less involves eating smaller portions and leaving the table when you might still feel hungry. That's what you need, certainly, but perhaps not what you really want. This week, choose not to complain about what you're sacrificing. God will give you exactly what you need each step of the way, and complaining stands in the way of recognizing His provision. If you get stuck in this mode, you'll have trouble hearing His voice of encouragement.

THE MIND FACTOR: GOT WORK ETHIC?

Recently my son Jake and I had a memorable mother-and-son conversation. It began with my asking him to clean the french doors in our living room. He complained and tried to get out of it. I didn't give in, and eventually he picked up the Windex and paper towels and slowly began the task. I think he was slightly worried that I might cancel his weekend fishing trip with his dad.

I paid close attention as Jake began the task with a slack attitude. He sprayed a little cleaning solution and moved his arm back and forth, investing minimum effort. As I watched, I could see that the glass was beginning to look even worse. Instead of criticizing him, I waited. A few minutes later I noticed that my son was beginning to take the job seriously. When he was finished, the doors looked great, and I was a proud mother.

As I sat down with Jake for a chat, I explained the value of having a good work ethic. I told him, "It means that you always do the very best job you can and you don't look for the easy way out, even if no one is watching and a fishing trip isn't on the line." The same level of commitment is needed to take back your body and your health. You do what's necessary even when you lose interest and even when no one is looking.

You're already nearing the halfway point of Phase 2. Keep putting in the time, concentration, and effort. Keep showing up each day. You will become more confident and comfortable every week.

As you begin Week 6, answer these three questions:

1. What motivates me to keep going?

   _____

   _____

2. In which areas of my life am I beginning to see improvement?

   _____

   _____

   _____

3. In which areas do I need to work harder?

   _____

   _____

   _____

Taking a regular inventory will remind you of how far you've come and will help you identify where you're falling short. One thing I know for sure: you no longer have the same outlook you had when you started! Always look ahead and pat yourself on the back for the small successes along the way.

THE EXERCISE EQUATION: TURN IT UP

This week you will do the same workouts as last week—five days of cardiovascular activity for thirty minutes each day, and two days of strength training. You should be getting more comfortable on the stability ball. I promise, if you're diligent, it will happen.

This week let's turn up the heat! Add some or all of these challenges to your workouts.

Day 1: Spend ten additional minutes doing your cardio at a consistent pace.

Day 2: Add one extra set of repetitions to five of your core exercises. (For more information on core training, see page 112 of *Never Say Diet.*)

Day 3: Add five minutes of serious intensity to your cardio exercise.

Day 4: Do the wall squats with this added challenge: for the last three repetitions of each set, hold the squatting position for thirty seconds longer.

Day 5: For your cardio today, switch things up. Go back to the list from Week 1, or try something completely different. You choose! The point is to add some variety to your workouts.

Weigh Yourself
Record your weight at the beginning of this week.

Week 6 starting weight: _____ (gain or loss of _____ pounds)

WEEK 6 STRENGTH TRAINING (2 Days, 20 Minutes per Session)

By recording your strength-training sessions, you have a place to reference your efforts, improvement, and peak moments. Be sure to add the challenges when you are ready to push yourself harder. (For descriptions of these exercises, see pages 115–24 in *Never Say Diet*.)

1. Bridge: 10 Reps, 2 Sets

Day 1: _____

_____

Day 2: _____

_____

2. Trunk Lift with Arm T: 10 Reps, 2 Sets

Day 1: _____

_____

Day 2: _____

_____

3. Alternating Hip Extension: 10 Reps, 2 Sets

Day 1: _____

_____

Day 2: _____

_____

4. Seated March: 10 Reps, 2 Sets

Day 1: _____

Day 2: _____

5. Seated Abdominal Walk Out: 10 Reps, 2 Sets

Day 1: _____

Day 2: _____

6. Seated Diagonal Reaches: 10 Reps, 2 Sets

Day 1: _____

Day 2: _____

7. Trunk Curl: 10 Reps, 2 Sets

Day 1: _____

Day 2: _____

8. Wall Squat: 10 Reps, 2 Sets

Day 1: _____

Day 2: _____

9. Wall Lunge: 10 Reps, 2 Sets

Day 1: _____

_____

Day 2: _____

_____

10. Wall Push-up: 10 Reps, 2 Sets

Day 1: _____

_____

Day 2: _____

_____

WEEK 6 CARDIO TRAINING

Complete thirty minutes of cardio exercises for five days this week, as you have in previous weeks. Record in the space provided what kind of cardio exercise you did and how it went.

Day 1 date/exercise/duration:

_____

How did it go?

_____

Day 2 date/exercise/duration:

_____

How did it go?

_____

Day 3 date/exercise/duration:

_____

How did it go?

_____

Day 4 date/exercise/duration:

_____

How did it go?

_____

Day 5 date/exercise/duration:

_____

How did it go?

_____

_____

THE FOOD FACTOR: THE MAGIC OF PROTEIN

The magic of protein is the ability it possesses to keep you satisfied. As you begin to pay close attention to the fuel you're giving your body, you also find out how your body reacts based on your choices. This week plan to eat some form of protein in the afternoon between lunch and dinner. Many people find that this is the time of day they struggle most with food. The scenario usually goes like this: you choose a great breakfast, you eat a healthy midmorning snack, then you consume a perfect lunch. And then you get busy. By dinnertime you have allowed yourself to go several hours without food, and your body starts to fight, wanting calories. This is where the entire day can be ruined for weight loss.

To help you overcome this, here are seven suggestions for afternoon snacks that contain protein. Try a few of them, and find one or two that you really like. Then stick with them each day.

Day 1: Apple slices with 2 tablespoons low-fat peanut butter

Day 2: 1 banana and 20 whole almonds

Day 3: Four thin slices turkey lunchmeat; 4 ounces or 1 cup blueberries

Day 4: 1 cup fat-free yogurt, 1 Kashi bar (Pumpkin Spice Flax is awesome.)

Day 5: Protein shake (1 scoop protein powder, 1 cup skim milk, 6 strawberries, 1 packet sugar substitute)

Day 6: 1 cup cottage cheese, 1 orange

Day 7: 4 ounces low-fat, low-sodium lunchmeat, ½ baked sweet potato

Week 6 Food Log

Just like last week, record *everything* you eat. Seeing it on paper helps you understand how much you're consuming, which foods keep you feeling full, and which ones deliver the most fuel.

Day 1: _____

_____

_____

Day 2: _____

_____

_____

_____

Day 3: _____

_____

_____

_____

Day 4: _____

_____

_____

_____

Day 5: _____

_____

_____

_____

Day 6: _____

_____

_____

_____

Day 7: _____

_____

_____

_____

Got Faith?

Doing the Hard Work Is Supposed to Be Hard

Scripture for the week: [Jesus said,] "If anyone would come after me, he must deny himself and take up his cross daily and follow me. For whoever wants to save his life will lose it, but whoever loses his life for me will save it."

—LUKE 9:23–24

Quote for the week: "The victory of success is half won when one gains the habit of setting goals and achieving them."

—OG MANDINO

Almost any day could be a *great* day if we started the morning by reading these verses about what it takes to follow Jesus. In fact, this command is so important that it's recorded in all four gospels. Jesus reminds the crowds that laying down their lives is the only way they can find true life. By denying ourselves in some way each day, we remember the sacrifice of our Savior.

Think about this: Jesus knows exactly how stressful your life is.

He knows the challenges you face. After all, He lived here and had to face the same pressures you do. And He wants to help you. The command He gives is as focused as anything you might have used in the past to guide your life. But Jesus' command is much more meaningful.

The Lord is telling us to stay off the merry-go-rounds we keep hopping on. He's telling us to give up our old habits. He offers the promise of *life*. "Whoever loses his life for me will save it" (verse 24). When it comes to your process of transformation, let God lead, and then follow closely behind Him.

THE MIND FACTOR: PARTY ALL THE TIME

I love parties! I love planning them and hosting them. Even better is going to them—probably because it's less work. My very favorite are birthday parties.

Regular celebrations keep life fun and give us something to look forward to. I hope you realize that celebrating the progress you're making in changing your life is just as important as celebrating a birthday. When I decided to lose two hundred pounds, I set my first serious goal in the second month of my journey. It was an ambitious goal: I wanted to lose one hundred pounds by my thirtieth birthday. At first I was losing more than two pounds a week. But after I set the new goal, the personal challenge was on. I had a serious goal to achieve and a big party to plan!

As we begin Week 7, it's your turn to set a goal. Make it doable but something you will have to work hard to accomplish. As you set your goal, also think about how you will celebrate.

THE EXERCISE EQUATION: FIND THE TIME

Finding time to exercise can be one of your biggest challenges. No matter what happens this week, you show up every day! I'm talking about the day you wake up not feeling so hot, and the day you have to make that big presentation at work, and the day your kid gets sick or has a big science project due, and the day before you leave on that big sales trip. Don't allow the inevitable crises to give you an out. Show up anyway, even if your workout that day is not as intense as on other days. You promised to tell yourself the truth always. So don't allow the daily interruptions of life to become a new excuse.

For Week 7 do your cardio exercises for five consecutive days, and continue with strength training twice a week. In addition, do the following extra-credit exercises.

Day 1: Add fifteen minutes to your cardio workout. Smile and do it with a winning attitude.

Day 2: When doing the seated marches, try to hold a bottle of water out in front of you with both hands while you complete each set. This will cause you to shift focus, helping you work on your balance.

Day 3: Today mix it up! Choose two different kinds of cardio, and do each for fifteen minutes.

Day 4: In addition to strength training, use your stability ball and a partner for the following challenge. At the end of your workout, face each other, step ten feet apart, and throw the ball back and forth for one minute straight. Repeat two more times.

Day 5: Make your intensity intense today! For every four minutes of your cardio, add one minute where you step it up and work until you are nearly out of breath. This is your first experiment with an interval session.

Weigh Yourself
Record your weight at the beginning of this week.

Week 7 starting weight: _____ (gain or loss of _____ pounds)

WEEK 7 STRENGTH TRAINING (2 Days, 20 Minutes per Session)

By recording your strength-training sessions, you have a place to reference your efforts, improvement, and peak moments. (For descriptions of these exercises, see pages 115–24 in *Never Say Diet.*)

1. Bridge: 10 Reps, 2–3 Sets
Day 1: _____

_____

Day 2: _____

_____

2. Trunk Lift with Arm T: 10 Reps, 2–3 Sets
Day 1: _____

_____

Day 2: _____

_____

3. Alternating Hip Extension: 10 Reps, 2–3 Sets

Day 1: _____

_____

Day 2: _____

_____

4. Seated March: 10 Reps, 2–3 Sets

Day 1: _____

_____

Day 2: _____

_____

5. Seated Abdominal Walk Out: 10 Reps, 2–3 Sets

Day 1: _____

_____

Day 2: _____

_____

6. Seated Diagonal Reaches: 10 Reps, 2–3 Sets

Day 1: _____

_____

Day 2: _____

_____

7. Trunk Curl: 10 Reps, 2–3 Sets

Day 1: _____

_____

Day 2: _____
_____

8. Wall Squat: 10 Reps, 2–3 Sets

Day 1: _____
_____

Day 2: _____
_____

9. Wall Lunge: 10 Reps, 2–3 Sets

Day 1: _____
_____

Day 2: _____
_____

10. Wall Push-up: 10 Reps, 2–3 Sets

Day 1: _____
_____

Day 2: _____
_____
_____

WEEK 7 CARDIO TRAINING

Complete thirty minutes of cardio exercises for five days this week, as you have in previous weeks. And don't forget to add the challenges described earlier in this chapter (see pages 56–57). Record in the space provided what kind of cardio exercise you did and how it went.

Day 1 date/exercise/duration:

_____

How did it go?

_____

Day 2 date/exercise/duration:

_____

How did it go?

_____

Day 3 date/exercise/duration:

_____

How did it go?

_____

Day 4 date/exercise/duration:

_____

How did it go?

_____

Day 5 date/exercise/duration:

_____

How did it go?

_____

THE FOOD FACTOR: HABITS TO LAST A LIFETIME

In a few weeks the nutrition part of your training is going to get a lot stricter. Occasionally I receive an e-mail that asks why I don't introduce the eating plan much earlier in the *Never Say Diet* program. While I understand the question, bear in mind that this program begins at ground level. Many of the women who have gotten fit and lost significant weight through this program came to it having had no experience in disciplined eating or exercise.

Part of what makes the *Never Say Diet* plan work is that you won't try to lose all the weight in a month. Instead you have chosen to become a better person in *all* areas—body, mind, and spirit. That is the big goal: to be the best person you can be. Weight loss becomes the by-product of this process.

As we work through Phase 2, keep up the disciplined eating habits you're beginning to develop. Make sure your breakfast delivers at least 300 calories. Listed below is another meal idea that is great for breakfast. (This could also be an afternoon snack.)

Buy several containers of nonfat yogurt to have on hand in your refrigerator. Fill a large storage container with healthy ingredients for a homemade topping to create a yummy parfait. Here are suggestions for the topping:

    1 package low-fat Bear Naked brand granola

    2 cups chopped nuts of your choice

    1 cup dried cranberries

    1 cup raisins

    1 cup raw coconut

Keep these ingredients in your cupboard with a teaspoon close by. When you're in a hurry, grab the yogurt, throw on two teaspoons of topping, and head out the door! As long as the yogurt is around 100 calories, the total for the healthy parfait will be about 250 calories. Find a few things for breakfast that you love and keep repeating them. You'll have a boring—but still yummy—meal.

Week 7 Food Log

Continue to record everything you eat. Also note the size of portions.

Day 1: _____

_____

_____

_____

Day 2: _____

_____

_____

_____

Day 3: _____

_____

_____

_____

Day 4: _____

_____

Got Faith? 63

Day 5: _____

Day 6: _____

Day 7: _____

Laugh It Off!

More Laughter Means More Fun

Scripture for the week: "When the LORD brought back the captives to Zion, we were like men who dreamed. Our mouths were filled with laughter, our tongues with songs of joy.... The LORD has done great things for us, and we are filled with joy."

—PSALM 126:1–3

Quote for the week: "Always bear in mind that your own resolution to succeed is more important than any one thing."

—ABRAHAM LINCOLN

What great things has God done for you lately? I am amazed at how He shows up in my life on a regular basis. There are times when I'm too ashamed to cry out to Him, but He never fails to take care of me.

Life has a way of tempting us to lose sight of God's love and care. Everyone has negative thoughts and feelings. You may feel you haven't accomplished enough, fast enough. Or maybe you're still beating yourself up about the past. Here's what I know for certain: God wants to free you from your past—no matter what happened. He wants to give you songs of joy.

In Week 8 don't hesitate to pray for more joy. Ask God to open your eyes to all the ways He cares for you. Ask Him to restore your joy.

THE MIND FACTOR: THINK *ROCKY* THEME SONG!

Phase 2 ends this week. You're almost halfway through the training program already. You should be feeling like a champ!

At this point you've seen the benefit of making commitments and establishing a foundation of discipline. You've been exercising five days per week, you've added strength training to your cardio workouts, you've kept a close watch on what you eat, you've shifted your eating habits (times of eating, size of portions, calorie content), and you've kept a focus on the big goal: becoming the best person you can be every day.

This is a huge change from your previous life, and you've done it in less than eight weeks. Close your eyes and hum the theme song from *Rocky*. Picture Sylvester Stallone doing roadwork and then ending the workout by running up the steps of the Philadelphia Museum of Art. At the top he stops, turns, and raises his arms in a gesture of victory. You remember the song. *Dah, dah, daaaah, dah...* It makes you feel like you can do this. You're a winner!

Along with celebrating your progress, you might be holding your breath, wondering if you are just one day away from repeating your old mistakes. When those thoughts enter your mind, replace them with a picture of where you were when you began this process two months ago. You knew you needed to establish disciplined rules and habits to live by. In just two months your life has already changed!

Has there been a day here and there when you did not feel like working out? Of course there has. Nevertheless, you showed up. Have you felt like you could be much nicer to your kids if you ate just one brownie? I'm guessing that might have crossed your mind. But you reached for an apple instead. You've found that there is power in pressing on and working toward your goal.

THE EXERCISE EQUATION: FOCUS ON CONSTANT MOTION

In a few days you'll get acquainted with the exercise plan for Phase 3. Since this is your last week with the ten exercises from Phase 2, let's perfect them. Remember that during strength training you should focus on constant movement.

Lots of movement equals:

- time efficiency—you're training more muscles at one time;
- greater fat-burning benefit—you're using more energy in the same amount of time;
- fun—movement is exciting when your adrenaline kicks in.

Weigh Yourself

Record your weight at the beginning of this week.

Week 8 starting weight: _____ (gain or loss of _____ pounds)

Week 8 Strength Training (2 Days, 20 Minutes per Session)

By recording your strength-training sessions, you have a place to reference your efforts, improvement, and peak moments. Be sure to add the challenges described in Week 7. (For descriptions of these exercises, refer to pages 115–24 in *Never Say Diet*.)

1. Bridge: 10 Reps, 3 Sets

Day 1: _____

_____

Day 2: _____

_____

2. Trunk Lift with Arm T: 10 Reps, 3 Sets

Day 1: _____

_____

Day 2: _____

_____

3. Alternating Hip Extension: 10 Reps, 3 Sets

Day 1: _____

_____

Day 2: _____

_____

4. Seated March: 10 Reps, 3 Sets

Day 1: _____

Day 2: _____

_____

5. Seated Abdominal Walk Out: 10 Reps, 3 Sets

Day 1: _____

_____

Day 2: _____

_____

6. Seated Diagonal Reaches: 10 Reps, 3 Sets

Day 1: _____

_____

Day 2: _____

_____

7. Trunk Curl: 10 Reps, 3 Sets

Day 1: _____

_____

Day 2: _____

_____

8. Wall Squat: 10 Reps, 3 Sets

Day 1: _____

_____

Day 2: _____

_____

9. Wall Lunge: 10 Reps, 3 Sets

Day 1: _____

_____

Day 2: _____

_____

10. Wall Push-up: 10 Reps, 3 Sets

Day 1: _____

_____

Day 2: _____

_____

WEEK 8 CARDIO TRAINING

Complete thirty minutes of cardio exercises for five days this week, as you have in previous weeks. However, continue to try to squeeze in some of the added challenges as directed in Week 7. Record in the space provided what kind of cardio exercise you did and how it went.

Day 1 date/exercise/duration:

_____

How did it go?

_____

Day 2 date/exercise/duration:

_____

How did it go?

_____

Day 3 date/exercise/duration:

_____

How did it go?

_____

Day 4 date/exercise/duration:

_____

How did it go?

_____

Day 5 date/exercise/duration:

_____

How did it go?

_____

THE FOOD FACTOR: TRY TO LEAVE THE KIDS AT HOME

Even under the best circumstances, grocery shopping can be a nightmare when you're trying to change the way you eat. Having children in tow can make it a horror show. So try to do your shopping alone or with a supportive friend.

It is sometimes a challenge to feel confident that you're making the right food choices. The good news and the bad news are the same: you will not make the best choices all the time. I found in the beginning of my Brain Change that narrowing down the foods I bought and knowing exactly where to find those items in the store were big helps.

For Week 8, maintain the same nutrition and dietary habits from Week 7. You should still be giving up something, whether it's sugar or processed junk food or something else. Also, continue to cut back on your portions. Reread Phase 3 in *Never Say Diet,* beginning on page 125, and begin to prepare accordingly. Since food is fuel, start a grocery list of the high-fuel foods that you most like to eat—and which require minimal preparation. Keep those foods on hand. (This is also the time to start thinking about your favorite restaurants. What can you order that will work with the program?)

By next week, you'll begin to eat five times a day. If this sounds like it might be difficult, don't allow it be. Just keep it simple. To begin to simplify your meal choices, fill in the lists that follow.

Fruits I like:

_____   _____
_____   _____
_____   _____
_____   _____
_____   _____

Vegetables I like:

_____   _____
_____   _____
_____   _____
_____   _____

Protein food (meats, eggs, cottage cheese, yogurt, etc.):

_____   _____

_____   _____

_____   _____

_____   _____

_____   _____

Carbohydrates (sweet potatoes, oatmeal, etc.):

_____   _____

_____   _____

_____   _____

_____   _____

_____   _____

Snacks (nuts, popcorn, sugar-free gelatin or pudding, granola
bars, etc.):

_____   _____

_____   _____

_____   _____

The negotiable stuff (cereal, cheese, tortillas, hummus, salad
dressings, etc.):

_____   _____

_____   _____

_____   _____

_____   _____

Week 8 Food Log

As before, write down everything you eat and the size of portions. Also, note which foods are becoming favorites and which meal choices are most convenient, simple to prepare, and highest in fuel.

Day 1: _____

_____

_____

_____

Day 2: _____

_____

_____

_____

Day 3: _____

_____

_____

_____

Day 4: _____

_____

_____

_____

Day 5: _____

_____

_____

_____

Day 6: _____

_____

_____

_____

Day 7: _____

_____

_____

_____

Make Food Boring

Weeks 9–12

It Only Takes a Spark

God Wants to Light Your Fire

> ***Scripture for the week:*** "For God is working in you, giving you the desire to obey him and the power to do what pleases him."
>
> —PHILIPPIANS 2:13, NLT

> ***Quote for the week:*** "Don't pray when you feel like it. Have an appointment with the Lord and keep it. A man is powerful on his knees."
>
> —CORRIE TEN BOOM

"In everything you do, stay away from complaining and arguing, so that no one can speak a word of blame against you.... Let your lives shine brightly before them. Hold tightly to the word of life" (Philippians 2:14–16, NLT). Those aren't my words, but I hope that on most days my life reflects those attitudes and commitments. This is the way the apostle Paul described the life of a believer and the ways in which such a life contrasts with what goes on in the world around us.

It's so easy to complain, even though we know God cares for us and provides everything we need. Can you imagine how God felt when He delivered the Israelites out of Egypt and had to listen to their constant complaining as they wandered through the desert? But in spite of their bad attitudes, God provided for them. As the verse says, do *everything* without complaining or arguing. Notice it doesn't say, "everything except cooking, scrubbing floors, and exercising." The work you're doing has a purpose. It is helping release you from bondage. Choose to be positive, even when a negative attitude seems to be the most natural way to react.

THE MIND FACTOR: BORING IS BEAUTIFUL

I once had a serious love affair with food, and I know that making it boring is a necessary and beautiful thing. When you make food boring—in contrast to enticing, a source of your security, or even a best friend—you feel a new sense of control. And realizing that you can now control the power that food used to have over you is absolutely refreshing!

If you're thinking that you don't really want food to become boring, repeat after me:

- I am now letting go of this powerful question: "When's the next meal?"
- I am letting go of the pressure that comes with "What will I serve for dinner?"
- I also release the emotional response of "What am I in the mood for this time?"

THE EXERCISE EQUATION: THIS IS WHEN THINGS REALLY COME ALIVE

Phase 3 is about taking yourself to a more serious level when it comes to your fitness. By now, you're working out regularly. To keep this going, you need to seek a *passion* for exercise. The cardio portion of the program switches to four days per week for thirty minutes each day, and the fifth day you will complete a twenty-minute interval session. In addition, you will add ten new strength-training exercises twice a week for thirty minutes. The more you are willing to push yourself past your comfort zone, the faster you will transform your body.

Weigh Yourself
Record your weight at the beginning of this week.

Week 9 starting weight: _____ (gain or loss of _____ pounds)

It's Measurement Time
First, copy your initial measurements from Week 1 and your second-round measurements from Week 5 in the space at the top of page 79. Then next to your old measurements, record this week's measurements. And next to that, calculate the difference between today and Week 1. Congratulate yourself on the progress you're making.

WEEK 9 STRENGTH TRAINING (2 Days, 30 Minutes per Session)

In this first week of Phase 3, you'll be learning new exercises for strength. They will be difficult at first, but soon you'll master them.

	Week 1	Week 5	Week 9	Loss or Gain (in inches)
Bust:	_____	_____	_____	_____
Chest:	_____	_____	_____	_____
Waist:	_____	_____	_____	_____
Hips:	_____	_____	_____	_____
Thighs:	_____	_____	_____	_____
Arms:	_____	_____	_____	_____

Continue to record your strength-training sessions so you'll have a place to reference your efforts, improvement, and peak moments. (For descriptions of these exercises, refer to pages 147–56 in *Never Say Diet*.)

1. Bridge with Hamstring Curl: 10 Reps, 1–2 Sets

Day 1: _____

_____

Day 2: _____

_____

2. Back Extension with Shoulder Blade W Squeezes: 10 Reps, 1–2 Sets

Day 1: _____

_____

Day 2: _____

_____

3. Side-Lying Leg Raises: 10 Reps, 1–2 Sets
Day 1: _____

_____

Day 2: _____

_____

4. Alternating Arm and Leg Raises: 10 Reps, 1–2 Sets
Day 1: _____

_____

Day 2: _____

_____

5. Push-up: 10 Reps, 1–2 Sets
Day 1: _____

_____

Day 2: _____

_____

6. Dumbbell Triceps Extension: 10 Reps, 1–2 Sets
Day 1: _____

_____

_____

Day 2: _____

_____

_____

7. Bent-over Dumbbell Row: 10 Reps, 1–2 Sets

Day 1: _____

_____

Day 2: _____

_____

8. Squat with Hammer Press: 10 Reps, 1–2 Sets

Day 1: _____

_____

Day 2: _____

_____

9. Diagonal Reach-ups: 10 Reps, 1–2 Sets

Day 1: _____

_____

Day 2: _____

_____

10. Side Lunge with Reach: 10 Reps, 1–2 Sets

Day 1: _____

_____

Day 2: _____

_____

WEEK 9 CARDIO TRAINING

Now that you're entering Phase 3, the cardio portion of the program switches to four days per week for thirty minutes each day. On the fifth day you'll complete a twenty-minute interval cardio session. (Find the details for the interval session on pages 131–33 of *Never Say Diet*.)

For Days 1–4 this week, continue the cardio workouts for thirty minutes each day as you have been doing in previous weeks. On the fifth day, complete the specified twenty-minute interval session. In the space provided, record what kind of cardio you did and how it went.

Day 1 date/exercise/duration:

_____

How did it go?

_____

Day 2 date/exercise/duration:

_____

How did it go?

_____

Day 3 date/exercise/duration:

_____

How did it go?

_____

Day 4 date/exercise/duration:

_____

How did it go?

_____

Day 5 date/(twenty-minute interval session):

_____

How did it go?

_____

The Food Factor: Eat Five Meals a Day

The number five looms large this week. Here's what it looks like to eat five meals a day:

> Breakfast
>
> Midmorning Snack
>
> Lunch
>
> Midafternoon Snack
>
> Dinner

Each of the five meals should supply 250 to 300 calories. If lunch is a little more than 300 calories, then cut back the midafternoon snack. In this program, we operate on calories, not a point system. Your decision at the beginning to "be interested" includes learning about calories and how to closely estimate a food's calorie content. In Week 9 you will continue to keep your food journal, but now add more detail as you try to include the calorie count whenever possible.

My Web site (www.chantelhobbs.com) has a calorie counter that will help you calculate a simple meal plan of 250 to 300 calories each. Once you calculate the calorie content in the main foods you eat, measuring the total for your meals will become simple. Start to estimate the calories in each meal by looking closely at labels. Pay attention to the total fat, saturated fat, and sugar content.

How to Organize a Week's Worth of Meals
- Create a list of three basic breakfast choices for the month.
- Make a list of six snacks for midmorning and midafternoon for the entire month.
- Make a list of three lunch selections (reread my story about the old standby, my fuel-packed turkey sandwich, on page 53 of *Never Say Diet*).
- Establish a list of five repeat dinners for the month.

Tip: Be sure to keep on hand the food you need for these five daily meals. When you do your grocery shopping, stock up on the staples.

Week 9 Food Log
Just as in Phase 2, write down everything you eat at each meal. The change this week is that you will eat smaller meals but more often (five times per day). Note the calorie content of each meal.

Day 1 date: _____

Breakfast: _____

_____

Midmorning snack: _____

_____

Lunch: _____

_____

Midafternoon snack: _____

_____

Dinner: _____

_____

Day 2 date: _____

Breakfast: _____

_____

Midmorning snack: _____

_____

Lunch: _____

_____

Midafternoon snack: _____

_____

Dinner: _____

_____

Day 3 date: _____

Breakfast: _____

_____

Midmorning snack: _____

_____

Lunch: _____

_____

Midafternoon snack: _____

_____

Dinner: _____

_____

Day 4 date: _____

Breakfast: _____

_____

Midmorning snack: _____

Lunch: _____

Midafternoon snack: _____

Dinner: _____
_____

Day 5 date: _____
Breakfast: _____

Midmorning snack: _____

Lunch: _____

Midafternoon snack: _____

Dinner: _____
_____

Day 6 date: _____
Breakfast: _____

Midmorning snack: _____

Lunch: _____
_____

Midafternoon snack: _____

_____

Dinner: _____

_____

Day 7 date: _____

Breakfast: _____

_____

Midmorning snack: _____

_____

Lunch: _____

_____

Midafternoon snack: _____

_____

Dinner: _____

_____

I Am Weak; He Is Strong

We Are Limited, but God Is Limitless

Scripture for the week: "Three times I pleaded with the
Lord to take it ["a thorn in my flesh"] away from me. But
he said to me, 'My grace is sufficient for you, for my
power is made perfect in weakness.'… For when I am
weak, then I am strong."

—2 CORINTHIANS 12:8–10

Quote for the week: "The grand essentials of happiness
are: something to do, something to love, and something to
hope for."

—ALLAN K. CHALMERS

Paul's statements about the thorn in his flesh will help you tap into
supernatural strength on your darkest days. Be encouraged and accept
that God's grace is sufficient for every situation, and best of all, He
never runs out of power! Think about how awesome it is that you
don't need to rely on your own limited strength.

No one knows suffering like Jesus. He not only faced the most horrible death we can imagine; it was undeserved. As the parable about sowing and reaping reminds us, we all will suffer consequences for sin even though we have received God's grace and forgiveness. However, when we struggle, God provides the strength to endure and complete the cleanup process. As you encounter challenges and struggles this week, use these verses from 2 Corinthians 12 to point you toward God's strength in your weakness.

THE MIND FACTOR: THIS IS PERSONAL!

I received a note from my son's third-grade teacher, asking me to attend a parent-teacher conference. I arrived and took a seat with my Dennis the Menace look-alike son. His teacher, Mrs. Wright, and another reading teacher assured me that my son's grades were excellent, his reading skills were above average, and so on. I was ready to run out and shout hallelujah!

Then both teachers paused. "Mrs. Hobbs, we have just one issue." One of the teachers said Jake has a tremendous amount of energy and can't sit still. He is always touching someone, jumping up, talking in class. *Surprise, surprise.*

Just when I was about to make my son apologize, he held up both hands and said, "So what you are saying is that I really shouldn't take all of this personally?" I dare you not to laugh. I had trouble avoiding it myself.

I reminded Jake that he was the person we were holding a conference to discuss, and, yes, he needed to take it personally!

How about you? Are you taking this program personally? If you're simply going through the motions, you run the risk of fizzling out. Remember: *you* know *you* need to lose weight, and *you* want to feel better about *yourself.* It can't get more personal than that.

THE EXERCISE EQUATION: THE SECRET OF BALANCE

Using the stability ball is fun and challenging. It forces you to do two things at once. You exercise, but you also must maintain your balance. It provides an enormous physical benefit.

I designed the strength-training program using the ball because I believe in the value of forced instability. Not only does it make you engage many muscle groups at once, but it's great mind training. When you think that the ball may roll away from you and that you won't be able to stay upright, a game begins. Tell yourself, "I can do three more reps…," and increase the challenge from there.

Weigh Yourself
Record your weight at the beginning of this week.

Week 10 starting weight: _____ (gain or loss of _____ pounds)

WEEK 10 STRENGTH TRAINING (2 Days, 30 Minutes per Session)

Continue to record your strength-training sessions so you'll have an ongoing history of your progress. (For descriptions of these exercises, refer to pages 147–56 in *Never Say Diet*.)

1. Bridge with Hamstring Curl: 10 Reps, 2 Sets
Day 1: _____

Day 2: _____

2. Back Extension with Shoulder Blade W Squeezes: 10 Reps, 2 Sets

Day 1: _____

Day 2: _____

3. Side-Lying Leg Raises: 10 Reps, 2 Sets

Day 1: _____

Day 2: _____

4. Alternating Arm and Leg Raises: 10 Reps, 2 Sets

Day 1: _____

Day 2: _____

5. Push-up: 10 Reps, 2 Sets

Day 1: _____

Day 2: _____

6. Dumbbell Triceps Extension: 10 Reps, 2 Sets

Day 1: _____

_____

Day 2: _____

_____

7. Bent-over Dumbbell Row: 10 Reps, 2 Sets

Day 1: _____

_____

Day 2: _____

_____

8. Squat with Hammer Press: 10 Reps, 2 Sets

Day 1: _____

_____

Day 2: _____

_____

9. Diagonal Reach-ups: 10 Reps, 2 Sets

Day 1: _____

_____

Day 2: _____

_____

10. Side Lunge with Reach: 10 Reps, 2 Sets

Day 1: _____

_____

Day 2: _____

_____

_____

WEEK 10 CARDIO TRAINING

For Days 1–4 this week, continue the cardio workouts for thirty minutes each day as you have been doing in previous weeks. On the fifth day, complete the specified twenty-minute interval session. (Find the details for the interval session on pages 131–33 of *Never Say Diet*.) In the space provided, record what kind of cardio you did and how it went.

Day 1 date/exercise/duration:

_____

How did it go?

_____

Day 2 date/exercise/duration:

_____

How did it go?

_____

Day 3 date/exercise/duration:

_____

How did it go?

_____

Day 4 date/exercise/duration:

_____

How did it go?

_____

_____

Day 5 date/(twenty-minute interval session):

_____

How did it go?

_____

_____

THE FOOD FACTOR: WHAT'S FOR LUNCH?

Because this month we're making food boring, I refuse to offer you yummy recipes. However, we'll get there eventually. Focus this week on your lunch choices. Without a solid lunch you can become ravenous late in the day. I don't want to hear that you aren't hungry enough to eat lunch or that you can't seem to find the time to eat. Remember, telling yourself the truth was the first of your Five Decisions.

Poor choices for your lunches makes it easy to fall apart for the rest of the afternoon. Before you know it, you're cramming Oreo cookies and Doritos into your mouth while pumping gas on the way home from work.

To avoid this, create a list that simplifies your meal planning and makes food boring. This week simplify your lunch planning by limiting your choices to three options. In the space below, fill in your three lunch options:

1. _____
2. _____
3. _____

Week 10 Food Log

Write down everything you eat at each meal. Remember, you're now eating smaller meals but more often (five times per day). Note the calorie content of each meal.

Day 1 date: _____

Breakfast: _____

_____

Midmorning snack: _____

_____

Lunch: _____

_____

Midafternoon snack: _____

_____

Dinner: _____

_____

Day 2 date: _____

Breakfast: _____

_____

_____

Midmorning snack: _____

_____

Lunch: _____

_____

Midafternoon snack: _____

_____

Dinner: _____

_____

Day 3 date: _____

Breakfast: _____

_____

Midmorning snack: _____

_____

Lunch: _____

_____

Midafternoon snack: _____

_____

Dinner: _____

_____

Day 4 date: _____

Breakfast: _____

_____

Midmorning snack: _____

_____

Lunch: _____

_____

Midafternoon snack: _____

_____

Dinner: _____

_____

Day 5 date: _____

Breakfast: _____

_____

Midmorning snack: _____

_____

Lunch: _____

_____

Midafternoon snack: _____

_____

Dinner: _____

_____

Day 6 date: _____

Breakfast: _____

_____

Midmorning snack: _____

_____

Lunch: _____

_____

Midafternoon snack: _____

_____

Dinner: _____

_____

Day 7 date: _____

Breakfast: _____

_____

Midmorning snack: _____

_____

Lunch: _____

_____

Midafternoon snack: _____

_____

Dinner: _____

_____

Jesus Loves a Little Patience

Don't Hold Back; Force Yourself to Have More

Scripture for the week: "And we pray this in order that you may live a life worthy of the Lord and may please him in every way: bearing fruit in every good work, growing in the knowledge of God, being strengthened with all power according to his glorious might so that you may have great endurance and patience."

—COLOSSIANS 1:10–11

Quote for the week: "Nothing great in the world has been accomplished without passion."

—G. W. F. HEGEL

Have you heard the saying "Patience is a virtue"? A virtue, according to Webster's dictionary, is a commendable quality or trait. I admit it—one of my major flaws is a lack of patience. I believe many of us are wired this way.

Like any skill or virtue, if it doesn't come naturally, you must practice it. At times I put something on my schedule that I don't like doing, simply because it forces me to practice patience. For example, taking a Pilates class bores me to tears. Yet I still show up (and on time!) because I know there is a great benefit in developing my patience. When the class is over, I'm never disappointed, but I'm still convinced that the clock was ticking in slow motion.

The best way to increase your patience is by choosing tasks that are challenging and that require a definite time commitment. Your cardio and strength training will often seem like impossible, time-consuming tasks. Practice patience by tackling them five days a week. Developing the virtue of patience will help in other areas of your life as well. Why not tackle a project you've been putting off, like cleaning out your garage? Or volunteering to teach the two-year-olds Sunday school class at church? Make sure the task requires patience and commitment. Then do it this week.

THE MIND FACTOR: REPETITION MAKES HABITS

Think about this: At their best, habits are the tools that keep us moving ahead in life. At their worst, they keep us stuck and miserable in negative, counterproductive patterns. But you have changed your brain, so you're done with the negative spiral. From now on, habits are one of the most powerful tools you have for becoming the best you can be.

At the beginning of Phase 3, I introduced you to the system of making food boring. This is necessary because old, unhealthy eating habits always try to creep back in. Eating one Girl Scout Samoa cookie sounds harmless, right? You can justify the calories by eating less for lunch or skipping your afternoon snack. However, here's the real issue. The discipline it takes for you to resist eating one cookie is the identical discipline required to fit in a workout on a really busy day.

Remember, we're telling ourselves the truth. Giving in to one cookie or piece of cake won't destroy us, but the truth is, it works against the powerful habit of patience that we need to develop. We are in this for *lasting results.* I want to hear stories of your long-term success for years to come. I want you to be fit and feel alive. To hit your target weight, the only cake you should contemplate for now is made with rice. Do you catch my drift?

If you want these same things, pay close attention: by making food boring, you can set aside certain foods that are exclusively for the occasional celebration. After practicing the virtue of patience, we can then feel free to celebrate when we have a legitimate reason for it.

THE EXERCISE EQUATION: WHY INTERVALS?

This week I'm going to introduce a new interval session for you to work into your cardio training. You will replace the usual twenty-minute session on Day 5 with the thirty-minute session as an added challenge this week. Remember why we do cardio exercise: it increases metabolic rate, reduces stress levels, increases alertness, improves digestion, and promotes a better immune system.

Weigh Yourself

Record your weight at the beginning of this week.

Week 11 starting weight: _____ (gain or loss of _____ pounds)

WEEK 11 STRENGTH TRAINING (2 Days, 30 Minutes per Session)

Continue to record your strength-training sessions so you'll have an ongoing history of your progress. (For descriptions of these exercises, refer to pages 147–56 in *Never Say Diet*.)

1. Bridge with Hamstring Curl: 10 Reps, 2–3 Sets

Day 1: _____

_____

Day 2: _____

_____

2. Back Extension with Shoulder Blade W Squeezes: 10 Reps, 2–3 Sets

Day 1: _____

_____

Day 2: _____

_____

3. Side-Lying Leg Raises: 10 Reps, 2–3 Sets

Day 1: _____

_____

Day 2: _____

_____

4. Alternating Arm and Leg Raises: 10 Reps, 2–3 Sets

Day 1: _____

Day 2: _____

_____

5. Push-up: 10 Reps, 2–3 Sets

Day 1: _____

_____

Day 2: _____

_____

6. Dumbbell Triceps Extension: 10 Reps, 2–3 Sets

Day 1: _____

_____

Day 2: _____

_____

7. Bent-over Dumbbell Row: 10 Reps, 2–3 Sets

Day 1: _____

_____

Day 2: _____

_____

8. Squat with Hammer Press: 10 Reps, 2–3 Sets

Day 1: _____

_____

Day 2: _____

_____

_____

9. Diagonal Reach-ups: 10 Reps, 2–3 Sets

Day 1: _____

_____

Day 2: _____

_____

10. Side Lunge with Reach: 10 Reps, 2–3 Sets

Day 1: _____

_____

Day 2: _____

_____

WEEK 11 CARDIO TRAINING

Just like last week, the cardio training is done on four consecutive days for thirty minutes each day. Consider mixing up which form of cardio you choose to complete. On the fifth day, use the interval session described below. For a reminder of the value of interval training, see pages 131–33 in *Never Say Diet*.

Day 5 Interval Training

Warm up for five minutes at intensity level 5 before beginning the thirty-minute interval session.

> Minutes 1–3, move from level 5 to level 6 as you begin to feel stronger.
>
> Minutes 4–10, maintain level 7.
>
> Minutes 11–15, reduce intensity down to level 4. Recover.

Minutes 16–20, work back up to level 8, minute by
minute.

Minutes 21–24, reduce work effort to a level 3. Take deep
breaths.

Minutes 25–26, work up to level 9. This is "press down on
the gas" time.

Minutes 27–28, recover down to level 2.

Minutes 29–30, go back up to level 5 where you started!

You need to gauge your intensity. It's important that you make
the most of all the intense work efforts. In the space provided, record
what kind of cardio you did and how long you maintained it per
session.

Day 1 date/exercise/duration:

_____

How did it go?

_____

Day 2 date/exercise/duration:

_____

How did it go?

_____

Day 3 date/exercise/duration:

_____

How did it go?

_____

Day 4 date/exercise/duration:

_____

How did it go?

_____

Day 5 date/(thirty-minute interval session):

_____

How did it go?

_____

THE FOOD FACTOR: DON'T DEHYDRATE

As you continue every day to eat five meals that deliver 250 to 300 calories each, be sure to drink plenty of water. Water plays a vital role by regulating body temperature, transporting nutrients and oxygen to the cells, removing wastes, cushioning joints, and protecting organs and tissues. Your body is made up of approximately 70 percent water. Each day you lose about two quarts through perspiration, urination, and breathing.

To make sure you're getting enough water, remember to use this formula: divide your body weight (in pounds) by two. This is the number of ounces of water you need to drink daily. (If you weigh 130 pounds, drink 65 ounces of water per day.)

Week 11 Food Log
Write down everything you eat at each meal, and note the calorie content of each meal.

Day 1 date: _____

Breakfast: _____

_____

Midmorning snack: _____

_____

Lunch: _____

_____

Midafternoon snack: _____

_____

Dinner: _____

_____

Day 2 date: _____

Breakfast: _____

_____

Midmorning snack: _____

_____

Lunch: _____

_____

Midafternoon snack: _____

_____

Dinner: _____

_____

Day 3 date: _____

Breakfast: _____

_____

Midmorning snack: _____

_____

Lunch: _____

_____

Midafternoon snack: _____

_____

Dinner: _____

_____

Day 4 date: _____

Breakfast: _____

_____

Midmorning snack: _____

_____

Lunch: _____

_____

Midafternoon snack: _____

_____

Dinner: _____

_____

Day 5 date: _____

Breakfast: _____

_____

Midmorning snack: _____

_____

Lunch: _____

_____

Midafternoon snack: _____

_____

Dinner: _____

_____

Day 6 date: _____

Breakfast: _____

_____

Midmorning snack: _____

_____

Lunch: _____

_____

Midafternoon snack: _____

_____

Dinner: _____

_____

Day 7 date: _____

Breakfast: _____

_____

Midmorning snack: _____

_____

Lunch: _____

_____

Midafternoon snack: _____

_____

Dinner: _____

_____

Stand Up, Stand Up to Temptation

Just Accept That It's Here to Stay

Scripture for the week: "The temptations that come into your life are no different from what others experience. And God is faithful. He will keep the temptation from becoming so strong that you can't stand up against it. When you are tempted, he will show you a way out so that you will not give in to it."

—1 CORINTHIANS 10:13, NLT

Quote for the week: "We first make our habits, and then our habits make us."

—JOHN DRYDEN

When I meet with a new client for the first time, I offer some suggestions on grocery shopping. Every time you go to the supermarket, it's easy to be tempted. So if you love potato chips, skip that aisle and don't even look down it. Same goes for the cookie aisle, the candy aisle, the soda pop aisle, and the in-store bakery.

Remember the story of Sodom and Gomorrah? God sent angels to tell Lot and his family to flee, warning them not to look back. Lot's wife ignored the warning, and after turning around for one last look, she turned into a pillar of salt (see Genesis 19:15–26). Looking leads to other things, so when it comes to food, spare yourself the temptation.

God will always give us a way out, but we shouldn't test Him by putting ourselves in a position that makes it hard to resist temptation. He will be faithful to you, but in a difficult situation it's easy for your desires to distract you to the point that you fail to call on Him for help. And trust me, it won't be God's voice you hear on the drive-through speaker at McDonald's saying, "May I help you?"

THE MIND FACTOR: START NEW RITUALS

"Night, night, Lukey. Go to bed. You are Mommy's little pumpkin head. Jesus loves you, and so do we, so close your eyes and go to sleep." I made up this song for my son when he was six months old. Now that Luke is five, the song has become a permanent part of our nighttime ritual.

If I am traveling, Luke has his daddy call me so I can sing to him over the phone. The song is as automatic as brushing teeth and saying prayers, and just as necessary. We need rituals because they give order to our lives and instill meaning in seemingly ordinary things.

Think about the steps you're taking to change your life. Then answer these questions:

1. Have you begun to implement new, healthy rituals? What are they?

_____

_____

_____

2. Is exercise becoming as routine as brushing your teeth? How did you make that happen?

_____

_____

3. Have you found a way to look forward to healthy yet boring food and eating healthy meals? If not, what is your biggest struggle in this area?

_____

_____

THE EXERCISE EQUATION: STRENGTH COMES FROM CHALLENGES

Think about the strength-training exercises, and name the ones that you prefer. As we come to the end of Phase 3, I want you to have confidence in your ability to start creating your own strength-training program. In addition to your exercises for the week, pick any two from Phase 2 each day—you can even vary which two—and add them to your scheduled workouts. Try to choose one that is easy for you and one that frustrates you like crazy.

Weigh Yourself

Record your weight at the beginning of this week.

Week 12 starting weight: _____ (gain or loss of _____ pounds)

WEEK 12 STRENGTH TRAINING (2 Days, 30 Minutes per Session)

Continue to record your strength-training sessions so you have an ongoing history of your progress. (For descriptions of these exercises, refer to pages 147–56 in *Never Say Diet.*) Remember to add two exercises from Phase 2 to your scheduled workouts each day. (For descriptions of exercises from Phase 2, refer to pages 115–24 in *Never Say Diet.*)

1. Bridge with Hamstring Curl: 10 Reps, 3 Sets

Day 1: _____

_____

Day 2: _____

_____

2. Back Extension with Shoulder Blade W Squeezes: 10 Reps, 3 Sets

Day 1: _____

_____

Day 2: _____

_____

_____

3. Side-Lying Leg Raises: 10 Reps, 3 Sets

Day 1: _____

_____

Day 2: _____

_____

4. Alternating Arm and Leg Raises: 10 Reps, 3 Sets

Day 1: _____

_____

Day 2: _____

_____

5. Push-up: 10 Reps, 3 Sets

Day 1: _____

_____

Day 2: _____

_____

6. Dumbbell Triceps Extension: 10 Reps, 3 Sets

Day 1: _____

_____

Day 2: _____

_____

7. Bent-over Dumbbell Row: 10 Reps, 3 Sets

Day 1: _____

_____

Day 2: _____

_____

8. Squat with Hammer Press: 10 Reps, 3 Sets

Day 1: _____

_____

Day 2: _____

_____

9. Diagonal Reach-ups: 10 Reps, 3 Sets

Day 1: _____

_____

Day 2: _____

_____

10. Side Lunge with Reach: 10 Reps, 3 Sets

Day 1: _____

_____

Day 2: _____

_____

_____

WEEK 12 CARDIO TRAINING

Do the cardio training four days for thirty minutes each day. On the fifth day complete the interval session for thirty minutes, as you did in Week 11. (You'll find the details for interval sessions on pages

131–33 of *Never Say Diet*.) In the space provided, record what kind of cardio you did and how it went.

Day 1 date/exercise/duration:

_____

How did it go?

_____

Day 2 date/exercise/duration:

_____

How did it go?

_____

Day 3 date/exercise/duration:

_____

How did it go?

_____

Day 4 date/exercise/duration:

_____

How did it go?

_____

Day 5 date/(thirty-minute interval session):

_____

How did it go?

_____

THE FOOD FACTOR: BERRIES—DO YOU KNOW HOW GOOD THEY ARE FOR YOU?

If you have ever had the pleasure of picking berries right from a garden or gathering wild berries, you know how delicious they can be. The most popular berries are naturally sweet and don't require much effort to prepare for eating. Just rinse and serve them.

Berries in general are a good source of vitamins and phytochemicals. Phytochemicals are components of fruits and vegetables that may help prevent certain diseases. For instance, blueberries and raspberries contain lutein, which is important for healthy vision. A cup of strawberries contains more than 100 milligrams of vitamin C, almost as much as a cup of orange juice. Berries are fabulous without anything added. But for a little flair, try serving a mixture of your favorite berries with nuts and just a touch of fat-free whipped cream.

Week 12 Food Log

Write down everything you eat at each meal, and note the calorie content of each meal.

Day 1 date: _____

Breakfast: _____

_____

Midmorning snack: _____

_____

Lunch: _____

_____

Midafternoon snack: _____

_____

Dinner: _____

_____

Day 2 date: _____
Breakfast: _____

_____

Midmorning snack: _____

_____

Lunch: _____

_____

Midafternoon snack: _____

_____

Dinner: _____

_____

Day 3 date: _____
Breakfast: _____

_____

Midmorning snack: _____

_____

Lunch: _____

_____

Midafternoon snack: _____

_____

Dinner: _____

_____

Day 4 date: _____

Breakfast: _____

_____

Midmorning snack: _____

_____

Lunch: _____

_____

Midafternoon snack: _____

_____

Dinner: _____

_____

Day 5 date: _____

Breakfast: _____

_____

Midmorning snack: _____

_____

Lunch: _____

_____

Midafternoon snack: _____

_____

Dinner: _____

_____

Day 6 date: _____

Breakfast: _____

_____

Midmorning snack: _____

Lunch: _____

Midafternoon snack: _____

Dinner: _____

Day 7 date: _____
Breakfast: _____

Midmorning snack: _____

Lunch: _____

Midafternoon snack: _____

Dinner: _____

PHASE 4

Get
Strong

Weeks 13–16

Let the Challenges Begin

It's Test-Taking Time

Scripture for the week: "Consider it pure joy, my brothers, whenever you face trials of many kinds, because you know that the testing of your faith develops perseverance. Perseverance must finish its work so that you may be mature and complete, not lacking anything."

—JAMES 1:2–4

Quote for the week: "Training gives us an outlet for suppressed energies created by stress and thus tones the spirit just as exercise conditions the body."

—ARNOLD SCHWARZENEGGER

Even if you've been out of school for years, you still have to take tests. And if you're like me, whenever you think about tests, you shudder as you go back to being in algebra class. You can still feel the dread you experienced when the teacher made the announcement. You remember the prayer asking God to help you get a passing grade.

Recently my daughter Ashley had to take a final exam for Spanish class. When it was over, I asked her how she did. "Okay, I guess," she said. Then she asked why it was necessary to take tests. I told her, "It's a chance to prove that you have learned the material and can remember it under pressure."

You've been taking a series of tests over the last three months. With each step and each small success, you have exercised your faith and developed perseverance. As you enter Phase 4, you have a chance to prove to yourself that you have changed.

THE MIND FACTOR: MAKE IT WORTH IT

As you start the fourth month, it's time to choose a meal for pure pleasure. It's fun to enjoy some of your favorite foods without guilt.

A few years ago I was invited to speak at a women's conference. The event coordinator called at the last minute, wanting to know if I believed in a "cheat day." I knew what she was asking: did I endorse a day to go off track? I explained that the words *cheat* and *cheater* are negative. They simply imply an inappropriate action.

So instead, think about it like this: after you have exemplified discipline, a celebration is in order! By integrating into your eating plan occasional foods that you don't eat on a regular basis, you will think of them as treats instead of part of your normal selections.

And that gets us to the test for this week: be sure to make this meal meaningful, just as you do the rest of the week's meals. Don't squander the calories on food that is average to your taste buds. Make it big!

The Exercise Equation: Let It Burn

Since I've been running marathons, a lot of people have told me they would love to run, but then they add, "I'm not really good at it." Boy, do I know the feeling! I can recall the first time I ran one mile on a treadmill. I could hear "We Are the Champions" playing in my head! From that point I began to build my endurance, one mile at a time.

It takes time to get good at becoming fit. But after you've been working at it this long, you can see real changes. After three months, you are a more fit person.

The exercises in Phase 4 are awesome for all-over toning. By adding free weights to your strength training, you'll feel a bigger burn during the exercise. It is essential that you force your muscles to work to the maximum. Pushing beyond your natural limits may create some soreness, so try to welcome it.

Weigh Yourself

Record your weight at the beginning of this week.

Week 13 starting weight: _____ (gain or loss of _____ pounds)

It's Measurement Time

First, copy your initial measurements from Week 1, your Phase 2 measurements from Week 5, and your Phase 3 measurements from Week 9 in the spaces below. Then next to your previous measurements, record this week's measurements. And next to that, calculate the difference between today and Week 1. Also, compare your Week 13 measurements with those of Week 9. Note the progress you made in the past four weeks, and don't forget to congratulate yourself!

	Week 1	Week 5	Week 9	Week 13	Reduction (in inches)
Bust:	___	___	___	___	___
Chest:	___	___	___	___	___
Waist:	___	___	___	___	___
Hips:	___	___	___	___	___
Thighs:	___	___	___	___	___
Arms:	___	___	___	___	___

WEEK 13 STRENGTH TRAINING (3 Days, 30 Minutes per Session)

For two days use the exercises listed below. On the third day create your own workout by drawing from the exercises in Phase 2, Phase 3, and Phase 4. For descriptions of those exercises, check the following pages in *Never Say Diet:* 115–24 for Phase 2, 147–56 for Phase 3, and 168–77 for Phase 4.

1. Bridge with Alternate Leg Lift: 10 Reps, 1–2 Sets

Day 1: _____

_____

Day 2: _____

_____

_____

2. Core Planks: 10 Reps, 1–2 Sets

Day 1: _____

_____

Day 2: _____

_____

3. Abdominal Crisscross: 10 Reps, 1–2 Sets

Day 1: _____

_____

Day 2: _____

_____

4. Ticktock: 10 Reps, 1–2 Sets

Day 1: _____

_____

Day 2: _____

_____

5. Jackknife: 10 Reps, 1–2 Sets

Day 1: _____

_____

Day 2: _____

_____

6. Biceps Curl: 10 Reps, 1–2 Sets

Day 1: _____

_____

Day 2: _____

_____

7. Chest Press: 10 Reps, 1–2 Sets

Day 1: _____

_____

Day 2: _____

_____

8. Standing Reverse Flys: 10 Reps, 1–2 Sets

Day 1: _____

_____

Day 2: _____

_____

9. Single-Leg Squat: 10 Reps, 1–2 Sets

Day 1: _____

_____

Day 2: _____

_____

10. Diagonal Chops with Knee Lift: 10 Reps, 1–2 Sets

Day 1: _____

_____

Day 2: _____

_____

_____

Day 3—Plan Your Own Workout

List the exercises from Phases 2, 3, and 4 that you're using in your own strength-training plan.

1. _____
2. _____
3. _____
4. _____
5. _____
6. _____
7. _____
8. _____
9. _____
10. _____

WEEK 13 CARDIO TRAINING

Do the cardio training four days for thirty minutes each day. On the fifth day complete the interval session for thirty minutes, as you did in Week 11. (You'll find the details for interval sessions on pages 131–33 of *Never Say Diet.*) In the space provided, record what kind of cardio you did and how it went.

Day 1 date/exercise/duration:

_____

How did it go?

_____

_____

Day 2 date/exercise/duration:

_____

How did it go?

_____

Day 3 date/exercise/duration:

_____

How did it go?

_____

Day 4 date/exercise/duration:

_____

How did it go?

_____

Day 5 date/(thirty-minute interval session):

_____

How did it go?

_____

THE FOOD FACTOR: MEAL PLANNING

The key word for meal planning this week is *simplicity.* I've tried fancy when it comes to meal preparation, but once I began my quest for healthier eating, I began to train everyone in my house that food isn't our top priority. When it comes to addressing our hunger, making the best choices *in an instant* is critical.

There was a day recently when I was famished, so I consumed every bite of a huge salad with chicken until I was positively stuffed. In that moment I had a life-changing thought about food: full is full. I feel as full after having a healthy salad as I would after consuming a Big Mac. So why do we fill ourselves on unhealthy food when we can eat clean and be just as full? It's often due to poor planning. If we plan better, we'll eat better.

This week make a list of ten healthy and balanced dinners that are simple to prepare. Once you've established this eating plan, go to the grocery store, and stock up on the needed ingredients. Always have these foods on hand. Then you can switch the combinations around for variety. Once a month try a new recipe so that everyone in your family has something to look forward to. You can even use one of the new recipes as one of your indulgence meals this week.

My Family's Top Ten Premium Meals

1. _____
2. _____
3. _____
4. _____
5. _____
6. _____
7. _____
8. _____
9. _____
10. _____

Week 13 Food Log

Write down everything you eat at each meal (five meals per day).
Note the calorie content of each meal.

Day 1 date: _____

Breakfast: _____

_____

Midmorning snack: _____

_____

Lunch: _____

_____

Midafternoon snack: _____

_____

Dinner: _____

_____

Day 2 date: _____

Breakfast: _____

_____

Midmorning snack: _____

_____

Lunch: _____

_____

Midafternoon snack: _____

_____

Dinner: _____

_____

Day 3 date: _____

Breakfast: _____

_____

Midmorning snack: _____

_____

Lunch: _____

_____

Midafternoon snack: _____

_____

Dinner: _____

_____

Day 4 date: _____

Breakfast: _____

_____

Midmorning snack: _____

_____

Lunch: _____

_____

Midafternoon snack: _____

_____

Dinner: _____

_____

Day 5 date: _____

Breakfast: _____

_____

Midmorning snack: _____

_____

Lunch: _____

_____

Midafternoon snack: _____

_____

Dinner: _____

_____

Day 6 date: _____

Breakfast: _____

_____

Midmorning snack: _____

_____

Lunch: _____

_____

Midafternoon snack: _____

_____

Dinner: _____

_____

_____

Day 7 date: _____

Breakfast: _____

_____

Midmorning snack: _____

_____

Lunch: _____

_____

Midafternoon snack: _____

_____

Dinner: _____

_____

More Praise, More Power

God Is More Satisfying Than an Ice Cream Sundae

Scripture for the week: "I will honor you as long as I live, lifting up my hands to you in prayer. You satisfy me more than the richest of foods."

—PSALM 63:4–5, NLT

Quote for the week: "The road to your championship will not be a smooth, wide and easily traveled freeway. No, great accomplishments are never realized without first having to endure steep climbs, hard falls and sharp turns."

—GREG WERNER

Anyone who has struggled with his or her weight knows the tremendous power of food. The verses from Psalm 63 acknowledge the food struggle as they describe the satisfaction of a rich feast. What I love most about this passage is that it uses food to help us remember where true satisfaction comes from. As we encounter the temptation to have the warm bread that is put in front of us at a restaurant or to answer the call of the cheesecake at a party, we can stop and think, *Do I need this? Can I praise the Lord instead and let Him satisfy my craving?* Submitting to Christ and offering Him a song of joy is the most gratifying thing in the world. As the words declare, "You satisfy me *more* than the richest of foods." When you are weak, by praising God you can find greater willpower than you have ever known!

THE MIND FACTOR: DO IT, THEN TALK!

Let me quote the now-famous words of my husband, Keith. When I told him I was going to lose two hundred pounds and then write a book about it, he said, "Chan, do it, then talk!" Now that you are fourteen weeks into your program, you are actually doing it!

This week as you celebrate how far you've come, start thinking into the future. Don't feel pressured to get all the weight off in a hurry or to start running marathons in a week. At the same time, I want you to recognize where you have been and where you are heading! You have bought a one-way ticket to freedom from low self-esteem.

Last week you enjoyed your first decadent meal in a long while. Now you should be feeling strong and in control. You are also not deprived; you are on fire! Be sure that you are burning with commitment to this process.

THE EXERCISE EQUATION: HOW TO CHOOSE THE RIGHT DUMBBELLS

Sometimes women are told to lift very light dumbbells to avoid gaining too much muscle mass. This advice is often taken to the extreme, and women perform too many repetitions using weights that are too light. Without sufficient load (weight), you won't see a significant change in the tone or shape of your muscles.

For shaping and toning, you must lift a weight that is heavy enough to create muscle fatigue (also known as failure). And don't worry that you'll end up looking like the Incredible Hulk. Even if you work your muscles to extreme fatigue, the majority of women are genetically unable to develop large muscles because they lack sufficient hormones or body structure. So do all the exercises this week with serious intensity!

Weigh Yourself

Record your weight at the beginning of this week.

Week 14 starting weight: _____ (gain or loss of _____ pounds)

WEEK 14 STRENGTH TRAINING (3 Days, 30 Minutes per Session)

For two days use the exercises listed below. On the third day create your own workout by drawing from the exercises in Phase 2, Phase 3, and Phase 4. For descriptions of those exercises, check the following pages in *Never Say Diet:* 115–24 for Phase 2, 147–56 for Phase 3, and 168–77 for Phase 4.

1. Bridge with Alternate Leg Lift: 10 Reps, 2 Sets

Day 1: _____

_____

Day 2: _____

_____

2. Core Planks: 10 Reps, 2 Sets

Day 1: _____

_____

Day 2: _____

_____

3. Abdominal Crisscross: 10 Reps, 2 Sets

Day 1: _____

_____

Day 2: _____

_____

4. Ticktock: 10 Reps, 2 Sets

Day 1: _____

_____

Day 2: _____

_____

5. Jackknife: 10 Reps, 2 Sets

Day 1: _____

_____

Day 2: _____

_____

6. Biceps Curl: 10 Reps, 2 Sets

Day 1: _____

_____

Day 2: _____

_____

7. Chest Press: 10 Reps, 2 Sets

Day 1: _____

_____

Day 2: _____

_____

8. Standing Reverse Flys: 10 Reps, 2 Sets

Day 1: _____

_____

Day 2: _____

_____

9. Single-Leg Squat: 10 Reps, 2 Sets

Day 1: _____

_____

Day 2: _____

_____

10. Diagonal Chops with Knee Lift: 10 Reps, 2 Sets

Day 1: _____

_____

Day 2: _____

_____

_____

Day 3—Plan Your Own Workout

List the exercises from Phases 2, 3, and 4 that you're using in your own strength-training plan.

1. _____
2. _____
3. _____
4. _____
5. _____
6. _____
7. _____
8. _____
9. _____
10. _____

WEEK 14 CARDIO TRAINING

Do four days of cardio for thirty minutes each day, and on the fifth day, complete your own personalized thirty-minute interval session—similar to the one you have been doing in Weeks 11, 12, and 13. Don't forget to record what kind of cardio you did and how long you maintained it per session. For a detailed description of interval training to use on Day 5, refer to pages 131–33 in *Never Say Diet*.

Day 1 date/exercise/duration:

_____

How did it go?

_____

Day 2 date/exercise/duration:

_____

How did it go?

_____

Day 3 date/exercise/duration:

_____

How did it go?

_____

Day 4 date/exercise/duration:

_____

How did it go?

_____

Day 5 date/(thirty-minute interval session):

_____

How did it go?

_____

THE FOOD FACTOR: PAY ATTENTION TO PORTIONS

We all love the feeling of conquering something! I believe that when it comes to food, this is why we tend to eat everything on our plates.

"Serving sizes in restaurants have gotten bigger," says Marion Nestle, professor of Nutrition and Food Studies at New York University. "Food is low in cost relative to rent and labor, so it's just as easy to throw in more food," and it's a tough thing to change.[3] This research explains one reason we tend to overeat. When people have become accustomed to large amounts, they feel cheated if the portion is reduced—closer to what it should be. The answer for you and me is simple: we must choose to eat less. And you can't leave this decision to the last minute. Before you take the first bite, decide how much you're going to eat, and save the rest for the next day.

Week 14 Food Log

This week monitor your portions closely and enjoy your special meal. Write down everything you eat at each meal, and note the calorie content of each meal.

Day 1 date: _____

Breakfast: _____

_____

Midmorning snack: _____

_____

Lunch: _____

_____

Midafternoon snack: _____

_____

Dinner: _____

_____

Day 2 date: _____

Breakfast: _____

_____

Midmorning snack: _____

_____

Lunch: _____

_____

Midafternoon snack: _____

_____

Dinner: _____

_____

Day 3 date: _____

Breakfast: _____

_____

Midmorning snack: _____

_____

Lunch: _____

_____

Midafternoon snack: _____

_____

Dinner: _____

_____

Day 4 date: _____

Breakfast: _____

_____

Midmorning snack: _____

_____

Lunch: _____

_____

Midafternoon snack: _____

_____

Dinner: _____

_____

Day 5 date: _____

Breakfast: _____

_____

Midmorning snack: _____

_____

Lunch: _____

_____

Midafternoon snack: _____

_____

Dinner: _____

_____

Day 6 date: _____

Breakfast: _____

_____

Midmorning snack: _____

_____

Lunch: _____

_____

Midafternoon snack: _____

_____

Dinner: _____

_____

Day 7 date: _____

Breakfast: _____

_____

Midmorning snack: _____

_____

Lunch: _____

_____

Midafternoon snack: _____

_____

Dinner: _____

_____

Keeping the Main Thing in Mind

Living a Balanced Life

Scripture for the week: "Be very careful, then, how you live—not as unwise but as wise, making the most of every opportunity, because the days are evil."

—EPHESIANS 5:15–16

Quote for the week: "Ability is what you're capable of doing. Motivation determines what you do. Attitude determines how well you do it."

—LOU HOLTZ

The only way to correct weakness is to be fully committed. The reward of following through on your commitment is the excitement of seeing results. In fact, after continued progress and the rush you get from pursuing even greater success, you can develop a compulsion that leads to an unbalanced life.

I once had an addiction to spinning. I decided to become an instructor, and before long I was accepting requests to teach classes everywhere in town. In a few months I was leading nine classes a week.

I came close to having a nervous breakdown. After many frank talks with my husband, I realized something had to give. I felt the Spirit of the Lord reminding me to keep Him first, then my family, then my fitness. It was hard to accept that the same compulsion that led to my eating an entire pint of ice cream in one sitting also caused me to exercise so much.

As you enter the next-to-the-last week of the Brain Change program, you should feel on top of the world. This could be the first time you've successfully lost weight and become fit. Paraphrasing the opening scripture, "Be careful how you live. Be wise and make the most out of every opportunity" (Ephesians 5:15–16). In other words, keep the main thing the main thing!

THE MIND FACTOR: ENERGIZE YOUR ATTITUDE WITH ACTION

"Whether you think you can or think you can't, you're right!" This quote by Henry Ford is one of my favorites. I want to get this message across: accomplishment is a direct result of your belief that anything is possible.

I know you've heard the saying "Attitude is everything." I propose a change: attitude is everything as long as it's backed up by action. People who decide to lose weight and get fit either make the necessary changes and maintain their fitness, or they eventually gain back the weight they lost. The factor that separates these two groups is the ability to keep acting on the commitment.

Match your good attitude with the necessary actions by finishing the following sentences:

I can _____

I can _____

I can _____

I can _____

I can _____

THE EXERCISE EQUATION: BUILD ON PAST SUCCESS

Ask yourself what you've learned about exercise so far. Do you feel better when you exercise? Do you realize that sweating is a great way to eliminate stress and toxins?

Last week I told you that muscle failure is important because it creates lean muscle and improves your metabolism. When you push your muscles during weight training, you'll have an increase in energy throughout the day, and you'll rest much better at night. By increasing your metabolism, you will burn more calories even when you're sleeping!

With a slow but steady increase in metabolism, it's possible for you to lose two to three pounds per week. The interesting thing about increasing your metabolism is that in order to burn calories, your body *needs* calories. Once you have limited your intake of calories to around 1,500 per day, cutting additional calories can slow down your metabolism to the point where you are no longer burning existing fat, and your body begins to store more fat.

Many fitness and weight-loss gurus have led the public to believe that aerobic or cardio workouts are the only effective way to lose weight. While they are important, they are not the be-all and end-all of weight loss. During your aerobic workouts, your metabolism does increase, and you burn more calories than you would if you were sitting on the couch watching television. But what happens when your workout is over? Your metabolism slows down. Your body is no longer burning extra calories. The key to increasing your metabolism is to build lean muscle so you will increase your metabolic rate while resting.

Weigh Yourself

Record your weight at the beginning of this week.

Week 15 starting weight: _____ (gain or loss of _____ pounds)

WEEK 15 STRENGTH TRAINING (3 Days, 30 Minutes per Session)

For two days use the exercises for Phase 4 listed below. On the third day create your own workout by drawing from the exercises in Phase 2, Phase 3, and Phase 4. For descriptions of those exercises, check the following pages in *Never Say Diet:* 115–24 for Phase 2, 147–56 for Phase 3, and 168–77 for Phase 4. Push past the pain and be intense!

1. Bridge with Alternate Leg Lift: 10 Reps, 2–3 Sets

Day 1: _____

_____

Day 2: _____

_____

2. Core Planks: 10 Reps, 2–3 Sets

Day 1: _____

_____

Day 2: _____

_____

3. Abdominal Crisscross: 10 Reps, 2–3 Sets

Day 1: _____

_____

Day 2: _____

_____

4. Ticktock: 10 Reps, 2–3 Sets

Day 1: _____

_____

Day 2: _____

_____

5. Jackknife: 10 Reps, 2–3 Sets

Day 1: _____

_____

Day 2: _____

_____

6. Biceps Curl: 10 Reps, 2–3 Sets

Day 1: _____

_____

Day 2: _____

_____

_____

7. Chest Press: 10 Reps, 2–3 Sets

Day 1: _____

_____

Day 2: _____

_____

8. Standing Reverse Flys: 10 Reps, 2–3 Sets

Day 1: _____

_____

Day 2: _____

_____

9. Single-Leg Squat: 10 Reps, 2–3 Sets

Day 1: _____

_____

Day 2: _____

_____

10. Diagonal Chops with Knee Lift: 10 Reps, 2–3 Sets

Day 1: _____

_____

Day 2: _____

_____

Day 3—Plan Your Own Workout

List the exercises from Phases 2, 3, and 4 that you are using in your own strength-training plan.

1. _____

2. _____

3. _____

4. _____

5. _____

6. _____

7. _____

8. _____

9. _____

10. _____

WEEK 15 CARDIO TRAINING

Do four days of cardio for thirty minutes each day, and on the fifth day, complete your own thirty-minute interval session. Record what kind of cardio you did and how long you maintained it per session. Be sure you stay challenged. In other words, as you become more fit, you may need to add intensity to get the same output of energy. For details of interval training, see pages 131–33 in *Never Say Diet.*

Day 1 date/exercise/duration:

_____

How did it go?

_____

Day 2 date/exercise/duration:

_____

How did it go?

_____

Day 3 date/exercise/duration:

_____

How did it go?

_____

Day 4 date/exercise/duration:

_____

How did it go?

_____

Day 5 date/(thirty-minute interval session):

_____

How did it go?

_____

THE FOOD FACTOR: DON'T FORGET FIBER

Because it can cause gas, bloating, and other uncomfortable side effects, fiber is easily ignored. However, research shows that a high-fiber diet may help prevent cancer, heart disease, and other serious ailments. So let's show roughage some respect! The typical American eats about fourteen to fifteen grams per day.[4] Health experts recommend a minimum of twenty to thirty-five grams of fiber per day for most people.

Week 15 Food Log

Continue to keep a written record of what you eat each day, including the high-fiber foods in your meals. Also, estimate the total calories for each of your five "meals."

Day 1 date: _____

Breakfast: _____

_____

Midmorning snack: _____

_____

Lunch: _____

_____

Midafternoon snack: _____

_____

Dinner: _____

_____

Day 2 date: _____

Breakfast: _____

_____

Midmorning snack: _____

_____

Lunch: _____

_____

Midafternoon snack: _____

_____

Dinner: _____

_____

_____

Day 3 date: _____

Breakfast: _____

_____

Midmorning snack: _____

_____

Lunch: _____

_____

Midafternoon snack: _____

_____

Dinner: _____

_____

Day 4 date: _____
Breakfast: _____

_____

Midmorning snack: _____

_____

Lunch: _____

_____

Midafternoon snack: _____

_____

Dinner: _____

_____

Day 5 date: _____
Breakfast: _____

_____

Midmorning snack: _____

_____

Lunch: _____

_____

Midafternoon snack: _____

_____

Dinner: _____

_____

Day 6 date: _____
Breakfast: _____

_____

Midmorning snack: _____

_____

Lunch: _____

_____

Midafternoon snack: _____

_____

Dinner: _____

_____

Day 7 date: _____
Breakfast: _____

_____

Midmorning snack: _____

_____

Lunch: _____

_____

Midafternoon snack: _____

_____

Dinner: _____

_____

Live Today Like It's Your Last

Making the Most of Every Moment

Scripture for the week: "Even youths will become exhausted, and young men will give up. But those who wait on the LORD will find new strength."

—ISAIAH 40:30–31, NLT

Quote for the week: "The legacy we leave is not just in our possessions, but in the quality of our lives."

—BILLY GRAHAM

I am so excited to share this news with you. Write this down somewhere and believe it: *I will win!* This is something you can count on! God has promised that if you trust Him, the victory is automatically yours.

The real question is, do you trust God? I challenge you to make this your mission each day from here on out. Trusting God is not a sometime thing; it's an everyday, all-the-time thing! The promise of new strength in Isaiah 40 is huge. Sure, we may have difficult days ahead, but check out the big picture. God will always be the greatest source of the strength we need to press on.

As you continue to run this race for life, prepare for success by beginning each day by surrendering to God. This will give you the victory every time.

THE MIND FACTOR: ROCK ON!

I would love to tell you that after I lost two hundred pounds, I never fluctuated a pound. That would be a lie. There will always be a range of about five pounds that you will teeter back and forth within. These pounds are the ones that creep on due to water retention, gain in muscle mass, or a little too much birthday cake and spinach dip at a party. Whatever the cause, stay on top of it. This means you shouldn't put your scale away for a month and then be surprised that you have gained some weight.

Keep the *Never Say Diet* program as a lifelong system. Because you have developed rituals, habits, and unconditional discipline over a period of months, it would be much more difficult to revert back to your old ways. Remember all five Brain Change decisions, and set out to be the best you can be each day.

THE EXERCISE EQUATION: SIX STEPS TO SUCCESS

Life gets crazy, and unexpected situations will always come up. That's why consistency is the major key to keeping physically fit.

Here are six tips to help keep your fitness on track!

Tip 1: Always keep two gym bags packed with the things you need for exercise. One bag you can take to work; the other goes in the trunk of your car. That way you'll always have workout clothes handy.

Tip 2: If you choose to work out in your home gym in the mornings, consider sleeping in your workout clothes. Then you will wake up ready to exercise!

Tip 3: At the beginning of each week, pledge that nothing that comes up will keep you from making your workout times happen!

Tip 4: Don't do the same exercises every time. You have more than sixty exercises at your fingertips in *Never Say Diet,* so make good use of them.

Tip 5: Workout buddies can be great, as long as you're not dependent on them. Ask a friend, your spouse, or one of your kids to join you for one workout a week! It's a great chance to spend time with someone you care about without using food as the reason.

Tip 6: You need duration for your workouts, but intensity is also important. Some days your schedule will allow for only a quick session. That's all right. Twenty minutes of an intense workout is far better than forty-five minutes of a mediocre one!

Weigh Yourself

Record your weight at the beginning of this week.

Week 16 starting weight: _____ (gain or loss of _____ pounds)

WEEK 16 STRENGTH TRAINING (3 Days, 30 Minutes per Session)

For two days use the exercises for Phase 4 listed below. On the third day create your own workout by drawing from the exercises in Phase

2, Phase 3, and Phase 4. For descriptions of those exercises, check the following pages in *Never Say Diet:* 115–24 for Phase 2, 147–56 for Phase 3, and 168–77 for Phase 4.

1. Bridge with Alternate Leg Lift: 10 Reps, 3 Sets

Day 1: _____

_____

Day 2: _____

_____

2. Core Planks: 10 Reps, 3 Sets

Day 1: _____

_____

Day 2: _____

_____

3. Abdominal Crisscross: 10 Reps, 3 Sets

Day 1: _____

_____

Day 2: _____

_____

4. Ticktock: 10 Reps, 3 Sets

Day 1: _____

_____

Day 2: _____

_____

5. Jackknife: 10 Reps, 3 Sets

Day 1: _____

_____

Day 2: _____

_____

6. Biceps Curl: 10 Reps, 3 Sets

Day 1: _____

_____

Day 2: _____

_____

7. Chest Press: 10 Reps, 3 Sets

Day 1: _____

_____

Day 2: _____

_____

8. Standing Reverse Flys: 10 Reps, 3 Sets

Day 1: _____

_____

Day 2: _____

_____

9. Single-Leg Squat: 10 Reps, 3 Sets

Day 1: _____

_____

Day 2: _____

_____

10. Diagonal Chops with Knee Lift: 10 Reps, 3 Sets
Day 1: _____

_____

Day 2: _____

_____

Day 3—Plan Your Own Workout

List the exercises from Phases 2, 3, and 4 that you're using in your
own strength-training plan.

1. _____
2. _____
3. _____
4. _____
5. _____
6. _____
7. _____
8. _____
9. _____
10. _____

WEEK 16 CARDIO TRAINING

Do four days of cardio for thirty minutes each day, as you have been
doing. Reserve the fifth day for your thirty-minute interval session.
Feel free to begin to mix in this interval session between Days 1 and

2 or Days 3 and 4 of your consistent cardio workouts. In the future, doing an interval session for your cardio every few days will help keep your body from getting used to the same workouts.

Day 1 date/exercise/duration:

_____

How did it go?

_____

Day 2 date/exercise/duration:

_____

How did it go?

_____

Day 3 date/exercise/duration:

_____

How did it go?

_____

Day 4 date/exercise/duration:

_____

How did it go?

_____

Day 5 date/(thirty-minute interval session):

_____

How did it go?

_____

The Food Factor: Your Nutrition from Now On

Repeat these statements about you and food:

- Food is fuel.
- Food has a job—to give me energy to do my life well.
- Food has never given me long-term happiness.
- Food has never solved a crisis in my life.
- Food will not take over my thoughts on a regular basis.

As you repeat these statements, it's important to understand each line and let it sink in. It's easy to become food obsessed by talking about food all the time. Let's face it: there are more important things in life.

Week 16 Food Log

By now you know the importance of keeping a written record of what you eat each day as well as the total calories.

Day 1 date: _____

Breakfast: _____

_____

Midmorning snack: _____

_____

Lunch: _____

_____

Midafternoon snack: _____

_____

Dinner: _____

_____

Day 2 date: _____

Breakfast: _____

_____

Midmorning snack: _____

_____

Lunch: _____

_____

Midafternoon snack: _____

_____

Dinner: _____

_____

Day 3 date: _____

Breakfast: _____

_____

Midmorning snack: _____

_____

Lunch: _____

_____

Midafternoon snack: _____

_____

Dinner: _____

_____

Day 4 date: _____

Breakfast: _____

_____

_____

Midmorning snack: _____

_____

Lunch: _____

_____

Midafternoon snack: _____

_____

Dinner: _____

_____

Day 5 date: _____

Breakfast: _____

_____

Midmorning snack: _____

_____

Lunch: _____

_____

Midafternoon snack: _____

_____

Dinner: _____

_____

Day 6 date: _____

Breakfast: _____

_____

Midmorning snack: _____

_____

Lunch: _____

_____

Midafternoon snack: _____

_____

Dinner: _____

_____

Day 7 date: _____

Breakfast: _____

_____

Midmorning snack: _____

_____

Lunch: _____

_____

Midafternoon snack: _____

_____

Dinner: _____

_____

Final Thoughts

I try not to let a day go by without thanking God for the opportunity to share with someone like you the immense passion I have for watching lives being transformed. The most rewarding result of my efforts is for you to catch a glimpse of the intense love that Jesus has for you. You are His beloved creation.

I used to be convinced that I was never good enough, but today I am joyfully free! Because God shows me His grace and mercy every day, I can tell you with confidence that it is possible to be free.

You have made tremendous progress over the past four months, so decide now that you will stay the course. Always strive to exceed your expectations. Create new challenges and peak moments along the way, and incorporate fun and memorable celebrations. Pledge not to allow old failures to dictate your future, and refuse to allow excuses to creep back in and take control of your life.

As you strive each day to be healthy, fit, and strong, remember that becoming the best you can be is a lifelong journey. I believe in you, but the best part is that God will always love you and believe in you.

Staying the course with you,

Chantel

(Contact me through my Web site at www.chantelhobbs.com.)

Notes

1. "Super Bowl Apparel Goes Global: Game Loss Is Win for Children and Families in Need," World Vision, January 25, 2008, www.worldvision.org/worldvision/pr.nsf/stable/2008 0125_superbowl.

2. Psalm 139:14

3. Marion Nestle, quoted in Bonnie Liebman, "Ten Tips for Staying Lean," *Nutrition Action Healthletter,* July 1999, http://cspinet.org/nah/7_99/ten_tips.htm.

4. American Dietetic Association, "Eat Fiber for Health," EatRight, September 22, 2004, www.eatright.org/cps/rde/ xchg/ada/hs.xsl/home_4033_ENU_HTML.htm.

This book is designed to be used along with Chantel Hobbs's book *Never Say Diet,* now available in paperback.

You can receive even more coaching from Chantel by visiting her Web site, www.chantelhobbs.com. Contact Chantel to find out how you can have her speak at your event. You can also download a free leader's guide to use with *Never Say Diet* and *The Never Say Diet Personal Fitness Trainer.* The leader's guide will help you get maximum results—plus shared support and encouragement—when you do the *Never Say Diet* program with other people. It works with any size group.

Also available at www.chantelhobbs.com is Chantel's cutting-edge online training program, which offers additional support to help you achieve lasting life change.

Chantel can be heard weekly on her radio program, *Facing Your Funk,* at www.ReachFM.org. Also, check out www.Made2Move Music.com, where you will find songs she recorded especially to get you movin'!

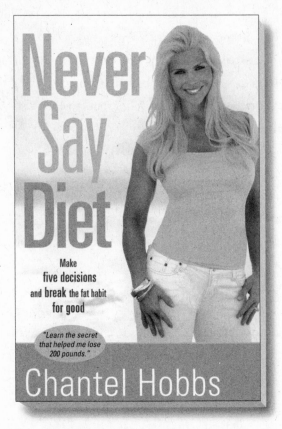
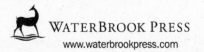